Implementing Eldercare Services

Implementing Eldercare Services

STRATEGIES THAT WORK

Ken Dychtwald
Mark Zitter
Joan Levison

McGraw-Hill Information Services Company

New York   St. Louis   San Francisco   Colorado Springs
Auckland   Bogotá   Caracas   Hamburg
Lisbon   London   Madrid   Mexico   Milan
Montreal   New Delhi   Panama   Paris   San Juan
São Paulo   Singapore   Sydney   Tokyo   Toronto

IMPLEMENTING ELDERCARE SERVICES
Strategies That Work

1234567890 DOC DOC 943210

ISBN 0-07-000533-8

This book was set in Century Book by the McGraw-Hill Book Com-
pany Publishing Center in cooperation with Monotype Composition
Company; the sponsoring editor was Deborah Glazer; the production
supervisor was Robert R. Laffler. The cover was designed by Alma
Orenstein. Project supervision was done by Harriet Damon Shields &
Associates. R.R. Donnelley & Sons Company was printer and binder.

Library of Congress Cataloging-in-Publication Data

Dychtwald, Ken, 1950–
   Implementing eldercare services : strategies that work / Ken
Dychtwald and Mark Zitter.
     p.   cm.
   Bibliography: p.
   Includes index.
   ISBN 0-07-000533-8
   1. Aged—United States—Health and hygiene. 2. Aged—United
States—Medical care. 3. Community health services for the aged—
United States. I. Zitter, Mark, 1958– . II. Title.
RA564.8.D93   1989
362.1'9897'00973—dc19   89-2766

Contents

2
Understanding and Marketing Eldercare 55

3
Eldercare Services 75

Preface

It is a trying time for America's health care industry. The government keeps ratcheting down payment rates even while it passes heightened quality of care legislation. Private insurers are negotiating tough contracts that squeeze profit margins and transfer financial risk to providers. Employers are demanding data on health outcomes, and consumers are doing everything possible to stay away from doctors and hospitals.

To top it off, America is aging at a rapid clip. Not only are Medicare reimbursement rates declining relative to costs, the systems and programs we have developed so successfully do not seem to be well suited for the burgeoning older population. For example, nearly a third of the older patients at our academic health centers contract iatrogenic illnesses, and an astonishing one-fourth of all hospital admissions for older adults are related to drug reactions or interactions. Less than one-fifth of one percent of our physicians are fully trained in geriatric medicine. Half of those in our nursing homes spend down to poverty before qualifying for government assistance. Even if providers could afford to care for older adults, can they do an excellent job at it?

There is some good news. Aging isn't what it used to be. Older adults as a group are far more healthy, active, independent, and financially self-sufficient than is commonly assumed—even by elders themselves. The National Institute of Aging tells us that 80 percent of health problems in the later years could be postponed or prevented entirely. Thus, the aging of America offers us all an unprecedented opportunity: the realistic possibility of living a long life filled to the end with health and vitality.

Whether or not America will take advantage of this remarkable opportunity will depend in large part on the energy and perspicacity of our health care leaders. Beleaguered as providers might be by the current health care environment, they must rise to an even greater challenge: the transformation of our established health care system into an *eldercare* system suited for the nation that we are becoming. If Americans over 55 will soon consume 75 percent of our health care resources, can providers have a more important challenge than eldercare?

If change is to occur, we must identify problems and create solutions. This book attempts to do some of each. Through a review of current social, economic, demographic, and health parameters of the older population and projections for the future, as well as statistics on health care utilization and how that usage is financed, we try to characterize the current state of affairs and pinpoint needed changes. Through descriptions of the strategic planning and marketing processes, financial feasibilities for individual eldercare services, and several case studies of leading eldercare programs, we focus on possible solutions. We intend this information, along with an explanation of the emerging eldercare system, to assist health care providers in managing the challenging business aspects of eldercare.

The companion book to this volume, *New Directions for Eldercare Services: Cooperation Along a Continuum,* provides a more detailed overview of the current and future population of older adults. In addition, that book includes information about the socioeconomics and health care utilization of older adults; suggestions for ways that providers might join forces with those organizations; and a description of the eldercare infrastructure so vital to accessing needed services.

The Directory of Information Sources at the end of this volume provides helpful access to the wealth of information available on aging. It includes extensive listings of associations, organizations, publications, and government agencies involved in the collection and analysis of these data. The List of Recommended Readings represents the tip of the iceberg. There are numerous excellent books and articles dealing with various issues of aging. The reading list is designed to act as an introduction into this particularly rich area of literature.

Older adults are not some isolated group for whom we feel sorry. They are our parents, grandparents, aunts, uncles, cousins, siblings, friends, and—currently or eventually—ourselves. We hope that this book and *New Directions for Eldercare Services: Cooperation Along a Continuum* will assist leaders in all fields in creating a health care system that enables all Americans to live their later years with health, independence, and meaning. Given the inexorable aging of America, we can have no higher priority.

Ken Dychtwald
Mark Zitter
Joan Levison

Acknowledgments

Books, like people, have lives of their own. And, as with human lives, book lives are touched and shaped by many individuals. Although the authors may serve as parents to a book, there are aunts, uncles, grandparents, cousins, and siblings who contribute to and support its birth and upbringing. Part of the fun of finishing a book is taking the time to thank publicly those people who have touched this effort and our broader lives.

We were fortunate to have a crackerjack team of researchers and writers contributing to our efforts. Joe Flower, Molly O'Lone, Galen Ellis, Malka Kopell, Connie Mahoney, and Cindy Wallace provided valuable research and writing support. We received additional help from Sue Adler, who is well on her way to becoming one of America's leading gerontological librarians, and from two others on the Age Wave research team, Judy Peck and Edith Fuller.

Our colleagues at McGraw-Hill also deserve our heartful thanks. Deborah Glazer's energy and insights helped shape the content and emphasis of this book. John Christoffersson and Lucigrace Koizumi also provided guidance and support.

Implementing Eldercare Services: Strategies That Work and *New Directions for Eldercare Services: Cooperation Along a Continuum* grew out of Age Wave, Inc.'s first premium report, *The Role of the Hospital in an Aging Society: A Blueprint for Action.* That publication is now the best selling report of its kind in health care industry history. We wish to thank here the many colleagues and friends, too numerous to mention individually, who contributed directly or indirectly to that highly successful work.

Finally, we wish to thank our families and friends. It is not easy living around people who write books, but those close to us seem to take our obsessions in stride and remind us by example of what is important in life. Sarai and Sam Zitter, Sherry and Robin Zitter, and Meryl Wolper were always there with their love and support. Monte Rosen, Steve Edelson, Scott Hecker, Jon Huggett, Ken Kannappan, Janice Bressler, Pete and Rebecca Hawthorne, Andrew Rich, and Mickey Levitan provide the friendship and love that is the stuff of life. Other blessings include Karen O'Callaghan, Don Wilcoxon, Paul and Heather Singarella, Liz Wilkerson, Margerie Nathanson, Paul Oxholm, Lisa Kirchoffer, Dave Richardson, Bonnie Karmiol, Gail Brady, Sheba Vegthe, Neil Steinberg, John and Dale Houck, Lynn and Bob Feeley, Susan Paterno, Mike DeLapa, Reva Gould, Betty and Steve Shagan, Glenn Evans, Marjorie Solomon, and Bill and Sue Gould.

Maddy Kent Dychtwald and Casey Kent Dychtwald bring the joy and love that makes life worth living. Pearl, Seymour, and Alan Dychtwald have never failed to support and nourish us in all our various endeavors and windmill chases. Stan, Sally, Richard, Linda, David, and Joel Kent as well as Frieda Gordet and Annea Neuss have become an unbeatable "second family." And last, who could ask for better friends and supporters than Jim Bernstein, Jean Duff, Fred Rubenstein, Michael and Alice Farmer, Bill Newman, Marc Michaelson, Diane Zinky, Jaymie Canton, Mark Goldstein, Joe Flower, Bruce Clark, Jeremy Tarcher, Peter Gottsegen, Morris Offit, Richard Schmeelk, Leonard Shaykin, and Gloria Cavanaugh.

About the Authors

Ken Dychtwald, Ph.D., psychologist, gerontologist, lecturer, and author, is a leading national authority on the social, life-style, and business implications of aging. As the chairman and chief executive officer of Age Wave, Inc., Dr. Dychtwald has consulted with and designed programs for a variety of corporations, health facilities, and government agencies. His publications include *Age Wave: The Challenges and Opportunities of an Aging America* (with Joe Flower); *Bodymind; Millennium: Glimpses into the 21st Century; The Keys to a Healthy Lifestyle; Wellness and Health Promotion for the Elderly;* and *The Role of the Hospital in an Aging Society: A Blueprint for Action* (with Mark Zitter); in addition to over one hundred articles in professional journals and magazines.

Mark Zitter, M.B.A., was until recently vice president of information services for Age Wave, Inc. His special expertise is in marketing to older adults, health care financing, strategic planning, and financial feasibility. A frequent contributor to professional and national publications, Mr. Zitter is also the author of *Marketing Healthcare to Older Americans* and coauthor of *The Role of the Hospital in an Aging Society: A Blueprint for Action* (with Ken Dychtwald). He holds guest lectureships at Stanford University and Yale Medical School. Mr. Zitter now heads the Zitter Group, a consulting and market research firm in San Francisco.

Joan Levison, M.B.A., is a principal of health care consulting services at Age Wave, Inc., where she is responsible for guiding health care institutions in strategic planning for and development of their eldercare programs and services. Ms. Levison directed the research which resulted in the publication of Age Wave's premium report, *Marketing Healthcare to Older Adults.* Her previous experience spans the fields of public and investor relations, insurance, and publishing.

Notes about
Data and Terminology

America has no central clearinghouse for information about health care and older adults. Although various branches of the federal government collect demographic and socioeconomic data about older adults, there is no source that maintains all, or even most, pertinent information about the fastest growing age segment of our society. Much information that could provide insight into the aging of America is not compiled by any office or organization. Thus, data collection and analysis represented a significant portion of the initial research involved in the preparation of this book.

A further problem with understanding the current older population is the age of the available data. Much important information, such as life expectancy or consumer spending, takes years to analyze, making the most recent figures somewhat dated. More problematic, some surveys are conducted infrequently (sometimes just once in a decade), further decreasing the relevance of the information to current planning. The data included in this report are the most current available as of November 1988.

All students of the aging of America have some trouble with terminology. The terms "elderly," "aged," "older persons," "mature adults," "elders," "older adults," "seniors," and "older Americans" often are used interchangeably. Some writers distinguish between the "young-old" and the "old-old," and others between "late adulthood" and "senescence." There even is disagreement over when "old age" begins, whether at 50, 55, 60, 65, 70, or beyond. Much of this muddle results from the vast diversity of the older population, and much of the linguistic anarchy is due to a lack of codification of the age groups.

Rather than confusing the situation further by creating our own definitions, we have chosen to use existing terminology to refer to the population in question. "Elders," "elderly," "older adults," "older persons," and "seniors," as well as several other terms, are used throughout this book. While most of our discussion is aimed at persons aged 65 and older, much is relevant to adults above age 50 or 55; this generally is obvious from the context. Similarly, when making distinctions within the older population, we occasionally use the terms "young old" and "very old," or "youngest old" and "oldest old"; the age breaks to which we refer should be implicit in the discussion. To the extent that we confuse our readers or fail to follow these guidelines, we apologize and hope that our ideas transcend the tangled terminology.

1

Demographics of Aging

The America of the past was a young nation. Aging and care for older people were not major issues in America at the beginning of this century because most people did not age; they died. According to the U.S. Census Bureau, in 1900 only three million Americans—one out of every twenty-five people—was over age 65. A baby born during that year could expect to live 47.3 years; the median age was 22.9. Only two-fifths of the population could expect to reach age 65, and the average 65-year-old would not reach 77.

Turn-of-the-century America was a youth-focused culture. Because over three-fourths of the population was under age 40, and since older people were scarce in both absolute numbers and relative proportions, social systems and structures were oriented predominantly toward the young. Why design facilities or create support programs for older people when disease or accidents killed the average person before he or she reached age 50? The young, especially that 45 percent of Americans below age 20, represented those with the greatest needs.

Old age in 1900 usually meant late fifties or early sixties. More than half of all people over 55 were under 65. Of those over age 65, nearly three-fourths were under 75. There were fewer than 125,000 people age 85 or more, representing just two-tenths of one percent of the total population. People over 65 accounted for only 4 percent of the entire population and only 7.6 percent of all adults.

As breakthroughs in medicine and public health allowed increasing numbers of Americans to live longer, the nation began to age, but the rate of change was moderate. By 1940, the number of Americans age 65 or over had tripled to nine million, accounting for 6.8 percent of the total population and 10.7 percent of all adults. A baby born that year could expect to live 62.9 years on the average—nearly 16 years longer than his father born four decades earlier. But most of the change in longevity was on the early end of life: more infants were living to adulthood. The relative age segments within the over-55 population had changed very little since 1900: more than half of that group still was below age 65, and more than 85 percent was under age 75. Old age had become somewhat more common, but very old age—at least, as we think of it—was still a rarity.

This gradual increase in the age structure of the population still had not captured the nation's full attention by the 1930s and 1940s. The country was preoccupied with the dramatic political and socioeconomic events of the times, including the Great Depression and World War II. Most of the over-55 population, and about half of those over 65, were still in the labor force; only one out of fifty Americans was over age 75. Thus, concerns about retirement and caring for the frail elderly were relatively mild.

Subsequent decades saw a dramatic rise in the older population. Between 1940 and 1970, the number of Americans over age 55 increased by 75 percent, while the number over age 65 more than doubled. By 1970, nearly one in ten Americans was over age 65. And now the older population itself was aging. The over-65 group now surpassed the 55- to 64-year-old segment in size, and the over-85 cohort had ballooned to nearly 1.5 million people, a 1200 percent increase since the turn of the century.

It was during this period that America finally began to notice its older people. President Harry S Truman called the first National Conference on Aging in 1950 to focus attention on the needs of older people. In 1961, the first White House Conference on Aging was held to make policy recommendations relating to older people. The Older Americans Act of 1965 established the U.S. Administration on Aging. That same year saw the passage of Medicare legislation designed to provide medical assistance for people over 65. Life expectancy reached 70 years. At last it was no longer unusual to attain old age.

America in the 1980s is an aging nation. The country's median age has increased from 22.9 years in 1900 to 31.8 years today. Our 29.2 million people over 65 comprise 12 percent of the population and one-sixth of all adults over the age of 21. Americans over 65 outnumber the total population of Canada. More than three-fourths of all Americans will reach their sixty-fifth birthdays; those who do have an even chance of living to reach age 82. A baby born today can expect to live for about 75 years. In July 1983, the number of Americans over 65 surpassed the teenage population. We are no longer a nation of youths.

Even the limits of old age itself have advanced. More than two-fifths of people over 65 have passed age 75. There are over three million Americans age 85 or over—25 times more than in 1900, and double the number in 1970. The 1980 census tallied 163,000 people over age 95 and more than 25,000 centenarians, a number that is projected to double in the 1990 census.

Because of this demographic upheaval, there has been increased attention focused on older people in recent years. The 1970s saw substantial expansion in funding for Older American Act programs and the establishment of state units and area agencies on aging (SUAs and AAAs, respectively) to coordinate their service delivery. The Federal Council on Aging was launched in 1974 to oversee federal programs for older Americans. The National Institute on Aging (NIA) was founded in 1975 within the National Institutes of Health (NIH).

Despite these important advances, it has been difficult for American policies and programs to keep pace with demographic realities. As a greater share of our population grows old, many support systems for older people are becoming overextended. A notable example is Medicare's hospital insurance (HI) trust fund, which is heading for insolvency in the mid-1990s, according to a 1986 report by the fund's trustees. This is due in part to rises in per capita health care costs, but also to unexpected increases in the number of eligible beneficiaries.

Why are we so out of phase with regard to the aging of our population? Partly because that aging has been so rapid. A rapidly evolving society is more likely than a static one to be out of step with its needs.

Figure 1-1 illustrates the dramatic growth of the older population in absolute terms during this century. The Census Bureau projects that the 29 million Americans over 65 in 1988 will become nearly 32 million in 1990 and nearly 35 million by the end of this century, accounting for nearly one-seventh of the population. During the last few decades, demographers have consistently understated

FIGURE 1-1
Population Over 55 Years by Age, 1900–1988

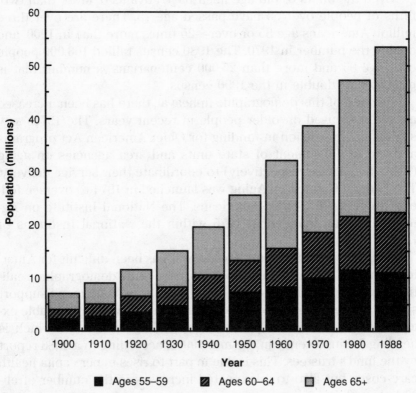

Source: Census Bureau, 1988

the number and proportion of older people in their projections, due primarily to unexpectedly low mortality and fertility rates.

The growth of the older population will accelerate again early in the twenty-first century as the postwar baby boom generation passes its mid-sixties. Robert Butler, former director of the National Institute on Aging, believes that people over 65 will account for as much as 20 percent of the population by 2020. The Population Reference Bureau projects that by 2025, Americans over 65 will outnumber teenagers by more than two to one. Five years later, in 2030, the nation's median age is projected to reach 41, according to the Census Bureau. As many as one in four Americans in the year 2050 may be over 65. Figure 1-2 depicts Census Bureau middle-series projections—those considered most likely to occur—of the number of Americans over age 55 for the next several decades, projections that many experts believe to be conservative. The aging of America, with all its challenges and opportunities, will continue through the middle of the twenty-first century, which is as far into the future as most demographers are willing to project.

What accounts for the changing nature of America's population structure? Americans are living longer and having fewer children. The increase in the *absolute number* of older people results from longer life expectancies and lower death rates. The rise in the *relative proportion* of older people is due to declining fertility rates.

Life Expectancy

Life expectancy is the average number of years a person of a given age can expect to live. Because mortality rates generally improve over time, projections of life expectancy usually understate people's actual survival prospects. Although the National Center for Health Statistics (NCHS) calculates life expectancies for every age through age 85, the most commonly cited statistics are life expectancy at birth and at age 65. An examination of the changes in these figures during this century sheds light on how and why our population has aged.

Life expectancy at birth already has increased by more than 27 years during this century. Census Bureau data show that a baby

FIGURE 1-2 _____
Projected Population Over 55 Years by Age, 1990–2050

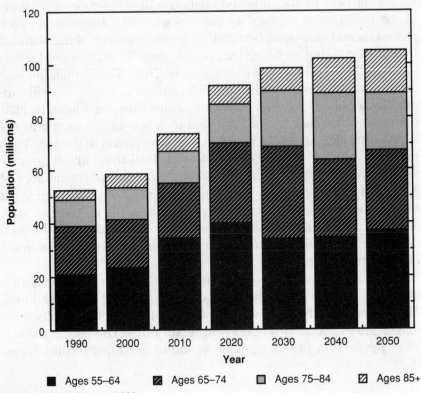

Source: Census Bureau, 1988

born today can expect to live nearly 75 years, compared with only 47.3 years in 1900. Much of this increase (20.9 years, or 77.1 percent) occurred by the year 1950. Due to improvements in sanitation and public health, and particularly to dramatic advances in the prevention and treatment of infectious disease, life expectancy at birth soared 44.2 percent during the first half of this century. Since then, life expectancy at birth has increased a modest 6.5 years (see Figure 1-3).

Much of the improvement in life expectancy at birth results from decreased infant mortality rates. Here, too, the largest gains oc-

FIGURE 1-3 _____

Average Life Expectancy at Birth by Sex, 1900–1986

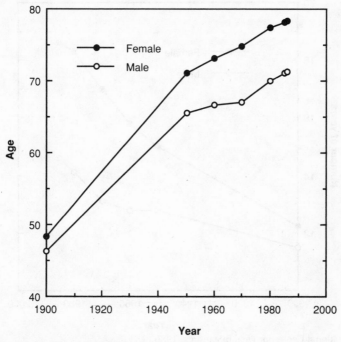

Source: National Center for Health Statistics, 1987

curred by 1950. At the turn of the century, 13.3 percent of babies born in the United States would not live to reach their first birthdays; 19.1 percent would not reach age 5. By 1950, those figures had plummeted to 3.1 and 3.6 percent, respectively. Since then, however, infant mortality rates have improved much more slowly: 1982 NCHS figures reveal that 1.1 percent of babies will not live a full year, and 1.4 percent will not reach age 5.

Since 1950, more of the gains in longevity have resulted from increased life expectancy at older ages. Life expectancy at age 65 has increased from 11.9 years to nearly 17 years during the twentieth century, but while 2 years were gained before 1950, 3.1 years already have been added since that year (see Figure 1-4). Recent gains are probably due to increased awareness of risk factors for

FIGURE 1-4

Average Life Expectancy at Age 65 by Sex, 1900–1985

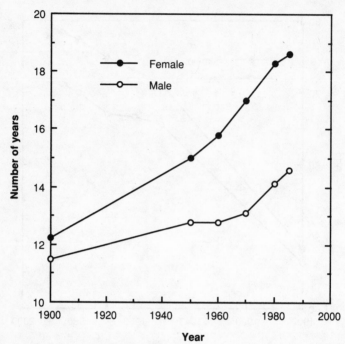

Source: National Center for Health Statistics, 1986

heart disease and cancer and to biomedical technologies that pro-
long the lives of patients who previously would have died. Thus,
since 1970, life expectancy at age 65 has increased nearly twice as
fast as life expectancy at birth (10.5 versus 5.4 percent).

Life expectancy is closely related to the population's age-
adjusted death rates (also known as mortality rates). *Age-adjusted
death rates* indicate mortality levels assuming no changes in the age
structure of the population from year to year. In 1985, the lowest
age-adjusted mortality rates in the nation's history were recorded:
546.1 deaths per 100,000 people. Although the figures were far higher
for older people—2838.6 deaths per 100,000 for the 65 to 74 group,
and just under 15,480 per 100,000 for those over 85—the Division
of Vital Statistics reports that every age segment experienced its

lowest death rate ever. Figure 1-5 shows the drop in death rates for older Americans since 1940.

The figures quoted above involve averages, which obscure many important subtleties. Life expectancy varies markedly by sex and race. On the average, women outlive men and whites outlive non-whites (although nonwhite women outlive white men). The latest available figures (NCHS, 1987) estimate life expectancy at birth for women at 78.3 years versus 71.3 years for men. This seven year difference seems to be decreasing slightly after peaking in 1979 at 7.8 years. Life expectancy at age 65 is four years higher for women than men (18.6 versus 14.6 years); the trend is similar to that of life expectancy at birth.

Up until the 1920s, life expectancy discrepancies between the

FIGURE 1-5

Age-Adjusted Death Rates for All Ages, 1940–1986

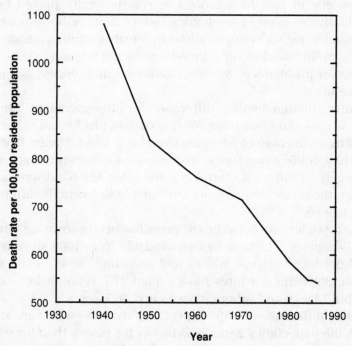

Source: National Center for Health Statistics, 1986

sexes were relatively minor: 1.8 years at birth and 0.5 years at age 65, according to the Social Security Administration. Since that time, the difference in life expectancy at birth has quadrupled, while the gap at age 65 has increased more than eightfold. Thus, most of the increase in the difference between male and female longevity can be attributed to declines in female mortality after age 65.

While the reasons for differences in life expectancy between men and women are not well understood, both biological and environmental factors exert an influence. Men tend to be involved in more stressful, dangerous, and physically demanding occupations and pursuits. Conventional wisdom posits that as women continue to choose careers and life-styles more similar to those of men, the longevity gap will diminish. But there is no evidence that this has occurred to any significant extent in the United States or other western countries, and few experts predict that the differential will decrease appreciably in the foreseeable future. Female mammals of other species tend to be longer-lived; the same may be true for humans, perhaps due in part to a protective role in health played by the reproductive system. Physiologists believe that the hormone estrogen, found in higher concentrations in females, inhibits plaque from building up in blood vessels, thereby reducing the incidence of cardiovascular problems in women. Cardiovascular disease is a major killer of men.

Similar, though smaller, differences in life expectancy exist between whites and nonwhites. Whites outlive blacks and other nonwhites by an average of 5.8 years from birth and 1.3 years from age 65. Although life expectancy discrepancies between the sexes are due largely to differing mortality rates *after* age 65, discrepancies between the races are primarily attributable to mortality differences *before* age 65.

The mortality gap between the races has been narrowing throughout this century. The best figures available from 1900 show a 14.6-year difference between whites and nonwhites in life expectancy at birth. Since then, whites have gained 27.7 years in life expectancy, but blacks and others have gained 36.7 years.

Racial differences in life expectancy dwindle with age, and by age 70, life expectancy actually is higher for blacks than for whites. This crossover effect may be due to high early mortality among blacks that leaves a relatively healthy older black population. Other explanations include racial differences in age-related health risk factors and protective factors in chronic disease. Mortality discrepancies between the races at younger ages are partly the result of differences in socioeconomic status; the mortality gap is unlikely to close until and unless income, housing, and education for blacks are improved.

Fertility Rates

While Americans have been living longer, they also have been bearing fewer children. The national fertility rate is less than one-fourth of what it was in 1800, having fallen by more than half between that year and 1910, and then again by half between 1910 and 1980. Since the late 1950s, birth rates among women of childbearing age have plummeted, from over 106 live births per thousand to under 66 per thousand. Today, America's population is growing for two reasons: high immigration rates and the baby "boomlet" caused by the unusually large number of baby boom women in their childbearing years. Were it not for these factors, the current birth rate of 1.8 children per woman would be insufficient to maintain population levels.

This long-term decline in fertility rates has occurred in all developed countries. Stanford University economist Victor Fuchs proposes three reasons for the trend: (1) a decrease in benefits of having children, (2) an increase in costs of raising children, and (3) a decrease in costs of avoiding having children. As industrialization has moved families from farms to cities and raised the age at which children begin working, children have become less useful to parents as producers and earners. As banks and social programs have evolved to provide for older people (or help them invest for their retirement), children have become less important as sources of insurance for later life.

The shift to an urban, industrialized society has also raised the costs of housing and feeding children. In recent years, the price of the mother's time in raising children—the dominant cost in child rearing—has risen as increasingly educated women have entered the labor force. Additionally, since expenditures per child are closely related to the family's living standard, improved life-style due to higher income has increased the average price per child.

Meanwhile, the cost of avoiding having children has dropped substantially. Contraception is cheaper, safer, easier, and more readily available than in the past. Also, the Supreme Court's decision supporting legal abortion in 1973 has facilitated the process of averting birth. According to the Center for Disease Control, in 1973, there were 19.6 abortions per 100 live births; by 1983, that figure had risen to 34.9.

Due to these and related reasons, fertility rates have declined steadily during the past two centuries, with the exception of the postwar baby boom (which was engendered by an unusual confluence of economic and social factors). Declining fertility leads to fewer young people relative to older people, assuming constant death rates. Mortality rates have not been constant, however, but have decreased as sharply as birth rates have fallen. These two demographic trends, decreasing fertility and declining mortality, have led to the dramatic rise in the population's age structure.

Substantial as these changes have been, they are likely to continue. Death rates probably will fall even further. Healthier life-styles and biomedical advances will continue to extend life expectancy, and many scientists believe that imminent research breakthroughs will allow us to slow the aging process itself. The outlook for fertility rates is similar: on the average, about 37 percent of 18- to 44-year-old women are childless. As a result, it is likely that the older population will continue to increase both in absolute number and relative proportion.

Just how much these trends will influence the population age structure is the subject of some disagreement. Variations in predictions of number and proportion of older people in future years result from difficulties in predicting changes in birth and death rates. Mortality rates are likely to be affected by technological advances and life-style modifications, both difficult to anticipate. Fertility trends will have a technological aspect, but will be more influenced by social patterns and, possibly, political action. For example, pronatalist policies recently have come to the fore in Europe, where some Eastern European countries have sharply curtailed access to legalized abortion. The only clear demographic consensus is that America will continue to age at an unprecedented rate.

Most Americans who are not yet 65 will reach that age, and those who do can expect to have many more years to live, barring unforeseen catastrophe. At the same time, however, older people have fewer children to rely on for emotional and financial support when needed. The aging of America thus generates a variety of new possibilities and problems, opportunities and burdens.

Age, Sex, and Race Characteristics

Aging of the Older Population

As noted earlier in this chapter, the age composition of the older group itself has increased markedly during this century. Figure 1-6 shows that, of all Americans over 65, the proportion who are over

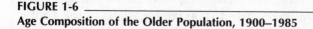

FIGURE 1-6

Age Composition of the Older Population, 1900–1985

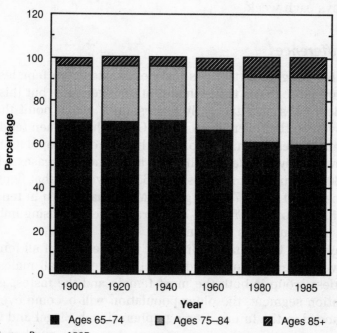

Source: Census Bureau, 1987

75 has ballooned from barely 25 percent in 1900 to more than 40 percent today. Of all Americans 55 and over, the proportion who are between 55 and 65 has dropped from 56.5 percent in 1900 to 44.7 percent today and will drop further, to a projected 34.5 percent by 2030.

Equally important, the over-85 group will continue to be the fastest growing population segment, increasing during the next 25 years from 1 to 2.4 percent of the total population and from 9.3 to 17.4 percent of the over-65 population. By 2050, according to Census Bureau projections, one in twenty Americans and nearly one-fourth of all people over 65, will be over age 85. This trend has profound implications for policymakers and health care planners, since geriatricians claim that serious health problems begin to appear most frequently between the eightieth and eighty-fifth years of life.

Finally, the ranks of the extremely old continue to burgeon. The 1980 census counted 163,000 people age 95 or above, compared with the 45,000 tallied in 1960. The Senate Committee on Aging reports that, as of 1988, there were over 45,000 centenarians in the United States, and more than 200 Americans celebrate their one-hundredth birthdays each week.

Sex Differences

Males have higher birth rates and death rates than females. Thus, there are more males than females at younger ages, but this difference decreases until the early forties, after which point there are more women than men at each age. Given that women tend to live longer than men, it is not surprising that the older population is disproportionately female and that the imbalance increases with age. Over 60 percent of Americans over 65 are women; that figure rises to 65 percent for the 75-plus group. More than seven in ten people over 85 are women. Figure 1-7 illustrates the increasing imbalance in age between males and females.

Looking at the situation differently, 14 percent of all females in 1984 were over 65, compared with 10 percent of all males. Since the oldest group is both the most female and the fastest growing population segment, the older population will become even more imbalanced in the future. Demographers Jacob Siegel and Cynthia Taeuber project that the discrepancy between the number of older

FIGURE 1-7 _____
Number of Males per 100 Females by Age Group, 1986

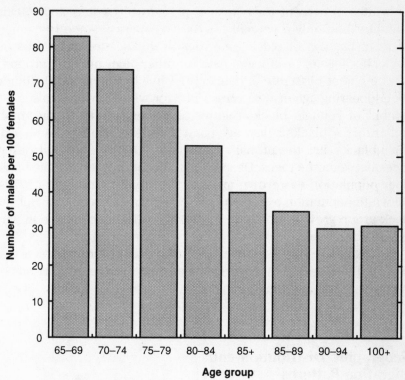

Source: Census Bureau, 1987

females and older males, now about 5.5 million, will grow to nearly 11 million by 2025.

Since most older people, particularly those over age 75, are female, the various problems associated with aging may be considered predominantly problems of women. Older women are often widowed and living alone, and they suffer from far higher disability and poverty rates than men of the same age.

Racial Differences

Just as life expectancy discrepancies among older people correspond to differing sex ratios, so do gaps between racial life expectancies lead to disproportionate race ratios. Nonwhites are underrepresented among older people. The Census Bureau reports that in 1982, the proportion of the population that was over 65 was about 12 percent for whites, 8 percent for blacks, 6 percent for Asians and Pacific Islanders, and only 5 percent for Native Americans and Hispanics. (Most discussion of older minorities in this section will focus on blacks because of insufficient data for other older minority groups.)

The higher birth rate of blacks (21.1 live births per 1000 women of childbearing age in 1985 versus 14.8 for whites), which raises the number of younger blacks relative to whites, and the higher mortality rate for blacks below age 65, which decreases the number of older blacks, are the primary reasons for the proportional differences between the races. Despite the current differences, the black elder population has grown much more rapidly. During the 1970s, the white population over 65 increased by about one-fourth, but the black group grew by about one-third. This difference is due in part to substantial gains in life expectancy experienced by blacks.

In the future, discrepancies in fertility and mortality rates are expected to increase the discrepancies between the proportions of the older white and black populations.

Geographic Distribution and Migration Patterns

Geographic Distribution

About half of older Americans live in eight states: California, Florida, Illinois, Michigan, New York, Ohio, Pennsylvania, and Texas. These are also the eight most populous states overall; of the group, only Florida and Pennsylvania have proportions of older residents significantly above the national average. Florida's 1986 figure of 17.7 percent over 65 is similar to that which the rest of the nation will experience in 2020. Florida also can claim to have the oldest population, with the median age being 36.0 years in 1986.

Recently, the southern states have become home to the largest portion of the nation's older citizens, with close to 10 million residents 65 and older. Between 1980 and 1986, the South and West experienced the most rapid increase in their older populations.

Three states led in the number of older immigrants between 1960 and 1980: Arizona experienced a 215-percent increase; Texas, a 191-percent increase; and Florida, a 110-percent increase.

It is apparent that every state will feel the impact of a growing proportion of older residents. However, the nature of the impact will depend on how each state's age structure shifts. Western and southern states, which are experiencing a net in-migration of older people, will need to erect and expand structures and programs to serve older people. On the other hand, many states in the Northeast and Midwest, which are losing younger residents to warmer climates, will experience smaller increases in their older populations, but will bear the burden of needy older people with a shrinking base of working-age residents.

Population Density

Most older people, like most Americans of all ages, live in cities. But this does not mean that urban populations are older than rural populations. To the contrary: the proportion of older people in a population varies in a rough inverse to its density—the more crowded the environment, the lower the proportion of old people.

Roughly 45 percent of the country's nonmetropolitan older people live in the South, while the Northeast and Midwest together account for only 25 percent. Three-fourths of the nonmetropolitan older people live in so-called small counties with towns no larger than 25,000. The 175 counties nationwide that had more than 20 percent of their populations over 65 in 1980 (including more than one-fourth of the counties in Kansas and one-fifth of those in Texas and Missouri) were usually small counties. Over half are located in the midwestern farm belt. However, many others fall within states with overall older proportions that are relatively small, such as Colorado, Georgia, Louisiana, New Mexico, and Texas. Thus, many areas, particularly rural and small town counties, may experience changes in their older populations that are contrary to broader regional trends.

Migration Patterns

Older people do move, but not as often as younger people. Propensity to change residences is highest for people in their early twenties. Americans over age 65 move from one house to another at less than half the rate of the general population. Only about 2 percent of people over 65 change their counties of residence in a year.

Migration of older people is nonetheless an important and growing demographic phenomenon. The number of interstate migrants over 65 rose from fewer than a million during the 1955–1960 period to over 1.6 million during 1975–1980. Nearly half of the movers over age 60 entered Arizona, California, Florida, New Jersey, and Texas. Other than New Jersey, which attracts New York City residents to its forests and seashores, the dominant migration pattern is out of the Northeast and Midwest and into the South and West. Retirement migration apparently is becoming increasingly common.

Although the trend appears to be changing, most of today's older people who move do not go far. Between 1975 and 1979, 78.3 percent of migrants over 65 moved within the same state, nearly three-fourths of those within the same county. Older people living within a city tended to move elsewhere within that city, while suburbanites stayed in the suburbs. Less than half of one percent of movers over 65 relocated from a suburb to the central city. People 55 to 74 were nearly three times as likely to move to a nonmetropolitan from a metropolitan area as the reverse; for people over age 75, migration was likely to occur equally in either direction. Overall, according to the Senate Committee on Aging, propensity to move among older people is greater for unmarried people and for those with higher levels of education; people in the labor force and those receiving assistance income are less likely to move.

A small but growing proportion of older people who move undergo a major relocation. Between 1975 and 1979, nearly 22 percent of migrants over 65 changed states, with two-thirds of them moving to noncontiguous states. Older people who change states tend to be affluent and well-educated relative to their peers. They often are accompanied by a spouse, and often have friends, family, or property in the new area.

In recent years, a pattern called *countermigration*—individuals over age 60 leaving the Sunbelt to return home—has arisen as a small but significant trend. During the late 1970s, nearly 100,000 people over 65 left Florida; approximately as many people over 65 left California as entered that state. Countermigrants are more likely to be older, widowed, and less educated than other older migrants.

It appears that many older people move as a result of a major life change, such as retirement or the loss of a spouse. In some cases, retirement may engender a migration to the South or West, and the subsequent death of a spouse may lead to countermigration back to the home state in order to be closer to children or old friends.

Housing

Home Ownership

Older people are more likely than the rest of the population to own their homes and to have paid off their mortgages. Of the 19.0 million U.S. households headed by people 65 years or older in 1987, 75 percent were owner-occupied; and 80 percent of those were completely paid off. Thus, over 60 percent of these households live mortgage- and rent-free. Surprisingly, two-thirds of all American homes owned free and clear belong to people over age 65.

Home ownership is most frequently associated with families, but more than one-third (36 percent) of over-65 owner-occupied houses in 1983 were inhabited by people living alone. The Census Bureau reports that renters are more likely than owners to live alone: about two-thirds of over-65 renters in 1978 lived by themselves.

Housing Condition and Cost

Although older people are more likely than the young to be home owners and to own their homes free and clear, older people also are more likely than other age groups to live in older homes, many of which are in poor condition. Among home owners in 1980, 70 percent of younger people but only 46 percent of people over 65 lived in homes built since 1950. These differences do not apply to renters.

Although older housing is not necessarily poorer housing, a relationship generally exists between a structure's age and its size, functional obsolescence, and ease of maintenance. The 1985 American Housing Survey reported that over 50 percent of people 65 and older live in units with severe or moderate physical problems and limitations.

Furthermore, housing problems of older people often differ from those of younger people: even houses in good condition are often too large or not suitable to current needs. Several studies have demonstrated that many older people live in homes too large for their current family size.

Housing costs vary greatly by ownership status, age, and sex. Home owners, younger age groups, and men tend to have lower housing costs as a percentage of household income. For example, the 1980 census found that housing costs averaged 10.9 percent of household income for men aged 65 to 69 who have paid off their mortgages, but 31.8 percent for women renters over age 85 and 39.3 percent for women over 85 who are still paying off their homes.

Housing expenses as a percentage of income rise with age because income is lower after retirement. The lowest expenses relative to income are incurred by men in their late fifties, who on average are enjoying their peak earning years.

Today's older people have available to them the widest variety of housing options in the nation's history. As the industry matures and the varied preferences of older people are better understood, housing options will continue to expand.

Boarding homes, traditionally open to persons of all ages, provide a bedroom, a private or shared bathroom, and a common dining area.

Congregate care retirement communities (CCRC) are housing developments planned, designed, and operated to provide a full range of accommodations and services for older adults, including independent living, congregate housing, and medical care. Residents move from one level to another as their health needs change. Typically, CCRCs require an entrance fee and monthly fees.

Congregate housing is specially planned, designed, and managed multiunit rental housing, with self-contained apartments. Services such as housekeeping, meals, transportation, and social activities are offered.

ECHO housing (Elderly Cottage Housing Opportunities) are self-contained, freestanding, temporary units adjacent to a single-family house. ECHO housing is designed for relatives of the home owners.

Foster care homes provide housing, meals, housekeeping, and personal care for nonrelated older adults.

Personal or residential care offers group living arrangements with staff-supervised meals, housekeeping, personal care, and private or shared bedrooms. Because of the level of care provided to residents, personal care facilities generally must be licensed.

Retirement communities are housing developments offering home ownership and rental units. Recreational and social activities often are offered, and support services are available on a fee-for-service basis.

Income, Wealth, and Spending Patterns

Popular descriptions of the economic status of older people are conflicting. According to prevailing stereotypes, older people are sick, lonely, and impoverished. Media coverage tends to focus on the economic plight of the widow struggling to survive on a fixed income. Senior political advocates lobby for funds to aid the sick and destitute.

At the same time, magazines targeted at older people lure advertisers by boasting of an affluent, fun-seeking population. Television shows such as *Dynasty* and *Love Boat* depict older people with money to spend. Luxury automobile manufacturers, cruise ship operators, and resort owners count on people over 55, and often over 65, for the vast majority of their revenues.

These conflicting images can result from the eagerness of various advocacy groups and marketers to depict older people in ways that support the particular cause being promoted. Magazines with older readers want advertisers to believe that those readers have the wherewithal to purchase luxury products. Journalists often find a good human interest story in the sick elderly couple whose government income subsidies are being cut. Yet the question remains: Are older people rich or poor? To answer this question requires exploring the income, wealth, and spending patterns of older Americans.

Income

Unquestionably, older people have lower average incomes than younger people. According to the Census Bureau, in 1987, the median cash income for families headed by people over age 65 was $20,813, far less than the $34,429 earned by families whose head was between 25 and 64 years old. Figure 1-8 illustrates that this gap increases with age.

Since families headed by older people on average are smaller than younger families, some income differential between the two is to be expected. The same pattern exists for unrelated people living alone or with nonrelatives. According to the Census Bureau, people over 65 not living in families earned a median of $7731 in cash income in 1986, less than half that of younger people not living in families, who averaged $16,880. Given that many in the latter group are single working people, this difference also is not surprising, but

FIGURE 1-8 _____

Median Income by Age of Household Head, 1987

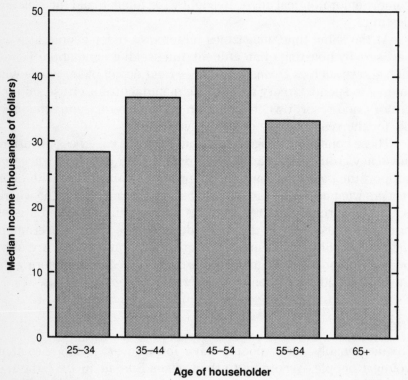

Source: Census Bureau, 1988

it does reveal how poorly older *single* people fare compared with younger singles.

Per capita income figures shed light on a different dimension. Census Bureau data show that people over 65 averaged slightly less per capita household income than the population as a whole and as much as or more than every age group except those in the prime earning years of 50 to 65.

Higher income levels among older people are related to marital status as well as age. Women who never married had the highest income of all women over 65, while married men had the highest income of all men over 65 ($8261 versus $12,666 in 1987). Married women had the lowest median income ($5485), but were likely to benefit from the earnings or pension of a male spouse; married men had the highest median income of any group ($12,666).

Although both age and marital status correlate with cash income, marital status is the better predictor for income level among older people. Single people are likely to have lower incomes than married couples, regardless of age. Evidence indicates that changes in marital status—which, for older people, usually mean the death of a spouse—are among the most important reasons for income decline among older people. This is to be expected for three reasons. First, a surviving dependent spouse receives just two-thirds of the Social Security benefits previously awarded to the couple. Second, if joint-and-survivor benefits are unavailable, pension annuities received by retired workers are forfeited upon death. Finally, when a working spouse dies, earned income is lost.

Since women are less likely to earn income than men and also tend to outlive their husbands, it is widowed women who have the most precarious economic position of any group. Widows had the lowest median income—$7432—of all women over 65 living alone in 1987, reflecting the loss of earnings or pension previously contributed by their husbands. Widowed women had a 1987 median income level nearly four-fifths that of widowed men.

Income among older people also differs by race. Older blacks and Hispanics have far lower cash incomes than their white counterparts; this is true for both sexes and at all ages. The Census Bureau reported that in 1987, whites over 65 reported a median income of $8975, while that of Hispanics was $5282 and that of blacks, $5081.

For white males over 65, median income was $12,398, whereas for Hispanics it was $6803 and for blacks it was $7167. For white females over 65, the median income was $7055; for Hispanic females it was $4526; and for black females it was $4494.

Poverty

Older people on average are slightly poorer than the rest of the adult population when measured by cash income, causing a higher proportion of older than younger people to fall near or below the poverty level.

Of course, the poverty level is a somewhat arbitrary definition of economic hardship. The picture appears worse for older people when this definition is broadened. Many more people over 65 than under 65 live *near*—defined as between 100 and 150 percent of—the poverty level (see Figure 1-9). In total, 29.1 percent of people

FIGURE 1-9 _____
Ratio of Income to Poverty Level for Elderly and Nonelderly Persons, 1987

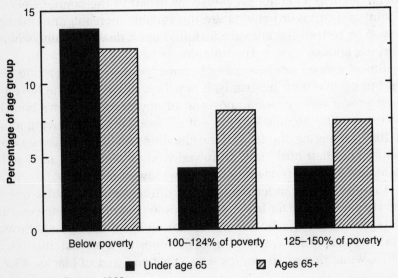

Source: Census Bureau, 1988

over 65 versus 24.3 percent of those under 65 lived below 150 percent of the poverty level in 1987.

The propensity to have incomes near or below the poverty level increases with age. According to the Social Security Administration, in 1986, 17.6 percent of the 85-plus group lived in poverty, compared with only 10.3 percent of those between 65 and 74. That same year, nearly one-third (30.6 percent) of the 85-plus group lived below 125 percent of poverty, but this was true for only one-sixth (16.5 percent) of 65- to 74-year-old people (see Figure 1-10). There is also a higher concentration of the oldest age groups at the lowest income levels.

Like many problems of older people, poverty is far more pervasive among women than among men. The low cash incomes of older women are primarily due to lifelong economic dependency on men and changes in marital status—usually widowhood—that occur in old

FIGURE 1-10
Ratio of Income to Poverty Level by Age, 1986

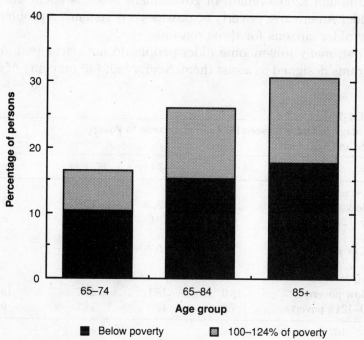

Source: Census Bureau, 1987

age. Census Bureau data show that the median income of women over 65 in 1987 ($6734) was just over half that of men ($11,854). Income for older men is higher than that of older women in every category of marital status. Table 1-1 shows that older women in all age groups are far more likely than men of the same age to be poor. Fifteen percent of women over 65 were poor in 1986 compared with only 8.5 percent of men. That year, women accounted for 59.6 percent of the population over 65, but 71.8 percent, or 2.5 million, of the poor.

Despite the prevailing notion that all older poor are supported primarily by government subsidies, a relatively small portion of older people below the poverty level rely on public funds for the majority of their incomes. In 1981, over one in seven persons over 65 were poor, but only one in nine received any cash income from public assistance. Of those who did, just one-third of them (one in twenty-seven persons over 65) received more than half of their income from public support. About 10 percent of the poor over 65 worked full time and year-round.

Although $269.5 billion of government funds is spent annually on older Americans, poverty or near-poverty remains a problem for many older citizens for three reasons.

First, many low-income older people do not participate in the programs designed to assist them. Nearly half (49 percent) of older

TABLE 1-1

Percentage of Older Persons by Ratio of Income to Poverty by Age and Sex, 1986

	65–74 yr	75–84 yr	85 + yr	Total 65 + yr
Both sexes				
Below poverty	10.3%	15.3%	17.6%	12.4%
100–124% poverty	6.2	10.6	13.0	8.1
Male				
Below poverty	7.0	10.7	13.3	8.5
100–124% poverty	5.2	7.5	9.6	6.1
Female				
Below poverty	13.0	18.1	19.7	15.2
100–124% poverty	7.0	12.6	14.7	9.5

Source: 1987 Current Population Survey

households below the poverty level received no cash or in-kind assistance from programs intended to aid the poor.

Second, the vast majority of funds spent on older people are not means-tested—that is, they are not awarded on the basis of a test of an individual's financial means—but go to social insurance programs and the like that are not income-based. In 1982, only 2.1 percent of the federal budget and about 8 percent of federal expenditures on Americans over 65 was spent on means-tested cash or in-kind transfers to the poor. In 1986, approximately four cents out of every dollar spent on people over 65 was expected to be used for means-tested programs such as Supplemental Security Income (SSI), housing, food stamps, and similar programs.

Finally, the largest means-tested programs, such as Supplemental Security Income, offer maximum benefits that are below the poverty level. Therefore, even those older people who receive maximum public assistance are likely to be poor even with the assistance.

Poverty rates for older people are substantially higher among minorities than among whites. According to the Census Bureau, the 1986 poverty rate for blacks over 65 (31 percent) was triple that of older whites (10.7 percent); the Hispanic poverty rate among people over 65 (22.5 percent) was double that of whites. Almost half (44.7 percent) of blacks over 65 lived below 125 percent of the poverty level. Minority women living alone had the highest poverty rates of any group; nearly three-fifths (59.3 percent) of older black women living alone had incomes below the poverty level in 1986.

Poverty levels vary by state, including relative poverty levels of people over and under age 65. According to the most recent available data, the poverty level among older people in most states was higher than the rate for younger people. The exceptions were New York, Florida, Arizona, and California; the latter three Sunbelt and western states tend to attract large numbers of relatively well-to-do retirees who raise the average income of older people.

The economic status of older people has improved markedly during the last several decades. The Census Bureau reports that in 1965, the median family income for families headed by people over 65 was $3460, less than half the $7537 average income of families headed by younger people. By 1987, older families had median incomes nearly two-thirds that of younger families ($20,834 versus

$34,429). During those two decades, income for people over 65 increased more than fivefold, while income of families headed by 25- to 64-year-olds rose less than four times.

This gain in income for older people relative to the rest of the population resulted from differences in sources of income. Younger people, most of whom are in the work force at any given time, suffered a decline in real income during the 1970s and early 1980s as the economy experienced several recessions. During that same period, older people enjoyed a steady rise in real income, based on growing Social Security benefits due to the retirement of generations with higher wage records. Meanwhile, automatic annual cost-of-living adjustments (COLAs) for Social Security benefits, introduced in 1975, kept the real benefits of those previously retired from declining. Thus, between 1977 and 1987, according to the Census Bureau, the median income of families headed by people over 65 increased in constant 1987 dollars from $17,099 to $20,834, while the income of younger families increased from $33,732 to $34,429.

Similar trends are evident in poverty rates. In 1959, more than one in three (35.2 percent) of all Americans over age 65 were poor—more than double the rate of younger adults (17.4 percent). Over the subsequent 15 years, average income for older people surged due to an overall rise in the standard of living and increases in Social Security and pension benefits. The most substantial gains in income levels of older people resulted from Social Security benefit increases in 1969 and 1972, COLAs from 1968 to 1971, and the 20 percent benefit increase included in the 1972 Social Security Amendments.

The effect of these factors on the economic status of older people was dramatic. The poverty rate for people over 65 was halved in just eight years, dropping from 28.5 percent in 1966 to 14.6 percent in 1974. During that same period, the poverty rate for younger adults decreased less significantly, from 10.6 to 8.5 percent, and it rose to 12.3 percent by 1982. By 1984, poverty rates for the two age groups were nearly equal (see Figure 1-11).

Affluence

Although older people have seen marked improvements in their economic status since 1960, they still earn lower median incomes than

FIGURE 1-11 _____

Poverty Rates for Nonaged and Aged, 1966–1986

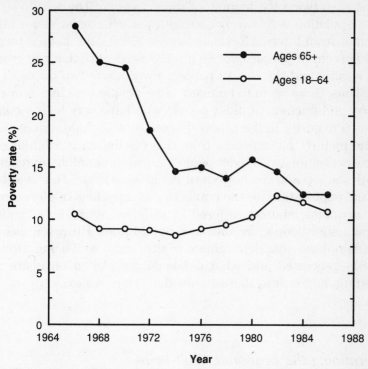

Source: Census Bureau, 1987

younger people and are disproportionately poor. However, not all older people are poor, and an increasing number are quite well-off. According to Find/SVP, a marketing information firm, 30 percent of all households with incomes exceeding $50,000 are headed by mature (over age 55) people. Mature households account for half of all luxury automobile purchases and spend far above the national averages for travel, alcoholic beverages, and dining away from home.

Households headed by people over 55 account for 30 percent of the nation's total personal income, nearly 80 percent of all money in savings and loan institutions, and 28 percent of all discretionary funds, compared with under 1 percent for people under age 25. Households headed by adults over age 55 own 25 percent of all automobiles and account for the majority of stockholders on the major and over-the-counter exchanges.

Much of the wealth of the over-55 population belongs to people under age 65 who are still in the work force. Adults between 55 and 64 earn twice the income of those over 65. The wealth of the older population is relatively concentrated: economist Victor Fuchs estimates from Internal Revenue Service (IRS) data that the wealthiest 1 percent of people over 65 hold 28 percent of that age group's total wealth, and the top 10 percent own nearly two-thirds of the total. Thus, there seem to be many older people who live in or near poverty and pockets of older people who have very high incomes, leaving a majority in the relatively comfortable middle range.

The picture that emerges from this discussion is a bimodal income distribution, with older people disproportionately represented at both the top and the bottom of the income scale. This is at least a partial explanation for the conflicting descriptions of older Americans' economic status proffered by different sources. In terms of income, older people are indeed rich and poor. However, cash income is not the sole determinant of economic well-being. How income is generated and what demands are placed on it are also important, and it is to these issues that we turn next.

Determining the Economic Well-Being of Older People

The preceding discussion paints a picture of the financial characteristics of the older population based solely on income. Yet cash income is a misleading measure of economic well-being for older people, for five reasons:

1. Older people have a different income mix than the young.

2. People over 65 have greater wealth than those under 65.

3. Older people receive more noncash benefits than younger people.

4. Much of the income flowing to older people is not taxed.

5. Older people receive several unique tax breaks.

Sources of Income

On average, people over 65 receive 40 percent of their income from Social Security and 25 percent from assets (see Figure 1-12). According to the Social Security Administration, as of 1986, only 12 percent of income for *aged units*—that is, a couple with at least one spouse over 65, or a person over 65 living without a spouse—was earned income.

In 1986, 91 percent of aged units derived some income from Social Security, and 15 percent of the 19,693,000 aged units receiving Social Security relied on it as the sole income source. Over one-third (34 percent) of aged units received more than 80 percent of income from Social Security. The poorest older people are most dependent on Social Security benefits: in 1982, aged units with incomes under $5000 received 77 percent of aggregate income from that source, compared with only 21 percent of aggregate income for aged units with incomes over $20,000.

FIGURE 1-12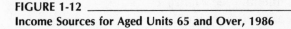
Income Sources for Aged Units 65 and Over, 1986

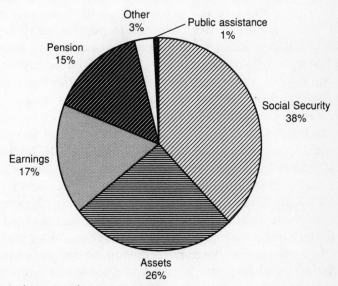

Source: Social Security Administration, 1987

Assets are another important income source for older people, accounting for a quarter of the income received by aged units in 1982. Income-producing assets include savings, rental property, investments, and various financial instruments. Income from assets has grown in importance to people over 65 during the past 25 years, rising from 16 percent of total income in 1962 to 22 percent in 1980. This income source is unevenly distributed: in 1986, 33 percent of aged units received no asset income, and 26 percent reported under $500 annual asset income. Only 33 percent of those receiving asset income garnered over $5000 a year from that source.

Earnings have the most substantial impact on the economic position of older people. Older people who work at full-time, year-round jobs have incomes similar to those of younger workers until age 70. In 1981, 41 percent of people 55 to 64 years old worked full time and year-round, compared with 10 percent of those between 65 and 69 and just 2 percent of people over age 70. The probability of continuing to work after reaching retirement eligibility is associated with the potential to earn more from work than from Social Security or pension payments (see Figure 1-13).

Employee pensions are another significant source of income for older people. Pensions provide 15 percent of income for people over 65. More than one in four (27 percent) aged units derived income from private pensions in 1986; another 16 percent received benefits from public pensions (either government employee pensions or railroad retirement). Because pensions are based largely on years in the work force, older men receive far more income from this source than does the current generation of older women.

The composition of income for older people has changed significantly during the past 20 years, largely due to rapid increases in real benefit levels during the late 1960s and early 1970s. In 1968, families headed by people over 65 received nearly half (48.2 percent) of their income from earnings and only 22.9 percent from Social Security. By 1983, earnings accounted for only 28 percent of income for these families, and Social Security had grown to 34.3 percent. The same patterns occurred for unrelated older people, although they tend to receive a much greater proportion of their incomes from Social Security. Figure 1-14 shows that earnings and assets increase in importance for older people with high money in-

FIGURE 1-13

Salary Replaced by Pension and Social Security after 40 Years of Work, 1986

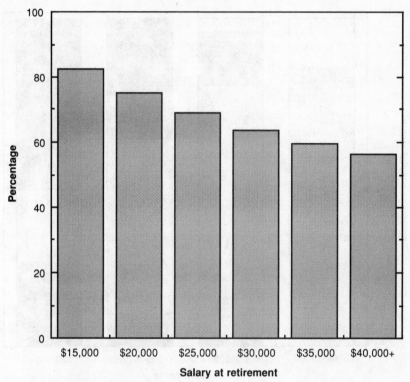

Source: Bureau of Labor Statistics, Employee Benefits Survey, 1987

comes, while Social Security payments and government assistance contribute proportionately more to income of poorer people.

Nonincome Determinants of Economic Well-Being

As a group, older people hold far more wealth than do younger people. People generally accumulate savings, real estate, and personal property during their lifetimes, so it is not surprising that older people have acquired more of such assets. However, as mentioned ear-

FIGURE 1-14 _____
Proportion of Total Money Income by Source for Persons Over Age 65, 1986

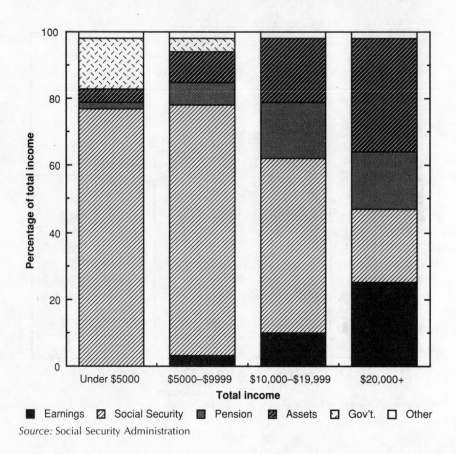

Source: Social Security Administration

lier, most controllable, transferable assets, such as real estate, securities, and savings, are concentrated in the hands of a few.

For many older people, the principal wealth held is in the form of home equity. In 1985, three-fourths of people over 65 owned their homes, and 83 percent of those had paid their entire mortgages. This equity is significant, but it is generally illiquid.

Another factor that confounds attempts to estimate the economic situation of older people involves in-kind benefits. Older people receive far more noncash benefits (such as Medicare and food stamps) than younger people. Nearly every person over age 65 is covered by Medicare hospital and physician insurance, which often have substantial value. Additionally, about one-fifth of households headed by people over 65 receive at least one of the various means-tested, in-kind benefits, including food stamps, public assistance housing, or Medicaid. Younger families also receive in-kind benefits not counted in income, such as group health insurance from employers, but these are proportionately and absolutely less substantial than the in-kind benefits received by older people.

Older Americans as a group have another economic advantage: they pay a smaller percentage of income in taxes than do younger people. Social Security, railroad retirement, and veterans' pension benefits are largely excluded from taxable income. All taxpayers over 65 enjoy a special exemption, and relatively low-income people over 65 receive a targeted tax credit. Also available is a one-time exclusion of capital gains from home sales beyond age 55. Finally, most older people pay no Social Security payroll tax. As a result, measures of pretax income tend to understate the relative financial condition of older people.

Given the difficulty in comparing the illiquid assets, noncash transfers, and tax advantages of older people to the earned cash income of younger people, what conclusions can be drawn about the relative economic resources of the different age groups? The consulting firm ICF, Inc., made the most ambitious recent attempt to address that issue in a study for the Milbank Memorial Fund in 1984, using 1980 data. Assets were valued as annuities, to be consumed at a steady rate over an individual's remaining life span, rather than as the imputed value of rent that the person would otherwise need to purchase. That analytic method was chosen to yield the higher income value for older people from assets so as to avoid biasing the results toward finding the old in poorer economic condition than the young. Adjustments were made for differences in levels of taxes and in-kind transfers.

Taking all these factors into account increased the apparent economic status of older people, but not quite to the level of those under age 65. With the inclusion of benefits and wealth, there were fewer people over 65 than under 65 below the poverty level (6.2 versus 9.8 percent). However, a higher percentage of people over

65 (32.5 versus 27.7 percent) remained below twice the poverty level (see Figure 1-15). Thus, noncash resources were more beneficial to older people than to younger people in 1980, but still did not compensate fully for differences in cash income.

Spending Needs and Patterns

Older people consume far more of their pretax income than do most younger households. The 1984 Consumer Expenditure Interview Survey conducted by the Bureau of Labor Statistics found that households in the youngest (25 and under) and oldest (65 and over) age categories consumed the highest proportions of their pretax incomes.

Older people spend primarily on necessities. Four-fifths of their

FIGURE 1-15 _____

Comparison of Economic Resources of Elderly and Nonelderly, 1980

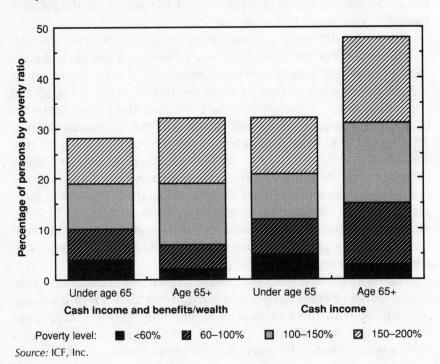

Poverty level: ■ <60% ▨ 60–100% ▨ 100–150% ▨ 150–200%

Source: ICF, Inc.

spending goes toward food, transportation, housing, and health care, compared with less than three-fourths of expenditures on those items by people 25 to 64 years old.

Differences in spending patterns are more closely related to income than to age. Thus, expenditures by workers over 65 do not differ significantly from those of workers in the 55 to 64 age bracket. Likewise, retired people under age 65 have spending patterns more similar to retired people over 65 than to workers in their own age group, according to Find/SVP, a market research firm. Apparently the needs and preferences of mature Americans are more closely related to work and income status than to chronological age.

Perspective on the Socioeconomics of Aging

The economic status of older people is far more complex than that of any other age group. Generalizing about the economic well-being of older people is complicated by three issues:

1. the high degree of variability within the older population,

2. the inadequacy of income as a measure of economic well-being, and

3. the difference in needs of older people compared with those of younger people.

The substantial economic gains that older people have realized have been achieved despite a significant reduction in the labor force participation of older men and the related drop in the proportion of income attributable to earnings for older households. Expansion of Social Security benefits and increases in pension and asset income made retirement more economically appealing to older people, many of whom responded by taking a portion of their rising living standard in the form of leisure. These phenomena are also largely responsible for the increasing numbers of people choosing to retire before age 65.

Thus, the answer to the question about the economic well-being of older people must be "It depends." On average, older people have a lower level of financial resources to draw upon than do younger adults. At the same time, they may have fewer financial demands than younger people (the exception being health care expenditures), and they accept—mostly by choice—a much larger share of their living standard in the form of leisure. On balance, studies have concluded that the economic status of older people has improved to the point where, upon retirement, they can generally maintain the standard of living enjoyed during their middle-age working years. The problem is that those with the greatest needs (especially in terms of medical care) may not be the ones with substantial resources.

In any case, it is possible to generalize about characteristics that are associated with wealth and poverty among older people. A typical poor older person is female, single, nonwhite, very old, and poorly educated, lives in a rural area, and relies largely on Social Security income. In contrast, wealthy older people are more likely to be married, white, under 75 years old, and living in a city or suburb; the bulk of their income is likely to come from physical assets, stocks, or earnings. These characteristics vary widely, with the best predictor of financial capability being marital status.

Prevailing attitudes about older people's economic well-being were formed before the legislative changes of the 1960s. At the start of that decade, one of three older Americans was poor—twice the poverty rate of younger adults. The introduction of Medicare and Medicaid, as well as an increase in Social Security and employer-sponsored pension benefits, has greatly improved the living standard of older people as a group. It no longer is accurate to think of most older Americans as poverty-stricken, nor is it reasonable to consider older people an affluent group. Older Americans are spread across the economic spectrum in a distribution even more diverse than the rest of the population.

Family Status and Living Arrangements

The last 25 years has seen a dramatic shift in the family status of older people, which, in turn, has influenced the living situations of older people. They are more likely to live alone than any other age group. Since people who live alone tend to be far more physically, emotionally, and financially vulnerable than those who live with others, these trends have serious consequences for the older population.

Marital Status

Differences between the sexes in marital status and living arrangements are profound. Women over 65 are more likely to be widowed (50.5 percent in 1986) than married (40 percent), and more than two-fifths (41.3 percent) live alone. In contrast, far more men over 65 are married (77.2 percent) than widowed (13.7 percent). There are at least three reasons for these differences between the sexes.

First, men are more likely than women to die at all ages, and this differential is particularly high late in life. At age 40 to 45, the death rate for men is 75 percent higher than the rate for women; at 50 to 55, it is 88 percent higher; and at 60 to 65, the gap peaks at 104 percent. Beyond age 65, the differential drops to 71 percent at 70 to 75 and 30 percent at 80 to 85.

The fact that women usually marry men older than themselves is a second reason for widowhood among older women. The likelihood that a woman will outlive her husband increases with age.

Another reason that older women are more likely than younger women to be without a spouse is that widowed or divorced men have much higher remarriage rates than do older women, and older men tend to marry women from younger age brackets. Divorce is more likely to occur earlier in life; between the ages of 45 and 64, divorced men have more than double the remarriage rates of divorced women. Widowed men over 65 have remarriage rates nearly seven times higher than those of widowed women.

Whatever the reasons for the relatively high number of widowed women, the disparity between the sexes increases with age. The differences between male and female marital status among older people have widened considerably during this century in correspondence with the increasing mortality gap (see Table 1-2).

This increase in widowhood for women relative to men indicates not a worsening problem for women but an improvement—that is, a reduction—in the incidence of widowhood for older men.

TABLE 1-2 _____
Ratio of Women to Men 65 and Older by Marital Status, 1900–1987

	1900	1920	1940	1960	1980	1987
Married	0.50	0.52	0.56	0.64	0.73	0.75
Widowed	2.21	2.14	2.33	3.31	5.34	4.98
Single	1.02	0.95	0.99	1.34	1.65	1.71
Divorced	0.57	0.53	0.58	1.06	1.30	1.43
All unmarried	1.97	1.86	1.90	2.61	3.84	3.66
All marital statuses	0.98	0.99	1.05	1.22	1.43	1.43

Source: Census Bureau, 1987

Living Arrangements

These changes in marital status among older people have been accompanied by concomitant shifts in living arrangements. The most prominent trends include a sharp rise in the proportion of women living alone and a decline in the proportion of men and women living with someone other than their spouses.

For the last 20 years, the proportion of men over 65 living alone has held fairly constant at about one in seven. In contrast, less than a third of women over 65 lived alone in 1965, but that figure surpassed 40 percent by 1984. The change has been even more dramatic for women over age 75, of whom 30 percent lived alone in 1965, and 51 percent lived alone in 1986. Widows and widowers are roughly twice as likely to live alone as to live with others. This phenomenon has increased rapidly: two-thirds of all widows lived alone in 1980, but less than one-fourth did so in 1950.

The increasing propensity of older women, especially the very old, to live alone, is projected to continue. By 1995, more than three-fifths of women over age 75 will live by themselves. The share of older men living alone is not likely to change significantly. The Census Bureau projects that by 1995, four-fifths of all people over 65 living alone will be women.

The share of men living with family members has hovered around 80 percent. Since 1965, however, older men have become much more likely to live with a wife than to be widowed and live with other family members. For both sexes, then, older people are less likely than in the past to live with other people after losing their spouses (see Table 1-3).

That a smaller proportion of older people are living with relatives is often considered a sign that family members are less willing to care for aging parents than in the past. This view has little basis in fact. Demographers Jacob Siegel and Cynthia Taeuber estimate that for every impaired nursing home resident, there are two equally disabled older people living with their families. Over one million American households include an older person needing help with basic activities or mobility, with as many as five million adult children providing care for their parents at any given time.

Historians point out that in western countries three-generation families have been relatively rare, largely due to the small number of people reaching old age. Although the *proportion* of older people living with their families has fallen, this is understandable for several reasons. First, longer life expectancies and declining fertility rates have increased the mother-to-daughter ratio (most often it is women who care for their elderly parents or parents-in-law).

TABLE 1-3

Living Arrangements of the Population 65 and Older by Age and Sex, 1970 and 1987

Living arrangement	Male			Female		
	65 + yr	65–74 yr	75 + yr	65 + yr	65–74 yr	75 + yr
1970						
In household	95.5%	96.4%	93.7%	95.0%	97.6%	91.1%
Living alone	14.1	11.3	19.1	33.8	31.6	37.0
Spouse present	69.9	75.2	60.4	33.9	43.5	19.1
With someone else	11.5	9.9	14.2	27.4	22.4	35.0
Not in household	4.5	3.6	6.3	5.0	2.4	8.9
1987						
In household	97.4%	97.6%	97.3%	97.7%	98.4%	96.8%
Living alone	15.6	12.3	21.8	40.9	33.5	51.5
Spouse present	74.9	79.7	65.9	39.2	51.0	22.4
With someone else	6.9	5.6	9.6	17.6	13.9	22.9
Not in household	3.8	2.1	7.1	6.3	2.2	11.7

Source: Census Bureau, 1988

Between 1950 and 1980, the ratio of women over age 65 to those between 35 and 44 doubled. It is new to the human experience that a majority of middle-aged women have living mothers: from 1940 to 1980, the proportion of 50-year-old women whose mothers were alive leaped from 37 to 65 percent.

Second, Americans have come to prefer autonomy whenever possible. As real income has increased, older people have had less economic motivation to double up with their children. Finally, failing health in old age has been a major reason that elders might move in with relatives or into nursing homes. Improvements in their overall health have allowed more older people to live independently, and increases in nursing home availability have made that option available to many who previously would have had no choice other than to live with relatives.

About 44 percent of households headed by someone over 65 consist of just one person; another 46 percent have two people. As noted above, most older people who live alone are women. However, it is not clear that living alone—at least as opposed to living with relatives—is associated with a lower quality of life for older people. Those living by themselves may be better off than those who have been forced to move in with relatives for health or economic reasons. Many older people living alone are not necessarily lonely and often have more outside contacts than people living with others. Women living by themselves tend to eat diets equally as nutritious as those eaten by married couples. This is not true for men, who may fare more poorly due to lack of experience in preparing meals.

Thus, there are four dominant trends in the living arrangements of older people:

1. an increase in older men and women who are married and living with their spouses,

2. a decrease in older people who are living with someone other than their spouses,

3. a rise in the proportion of older women who live alone, and

4. an increase in the proportion of households headed by older people that are maintained by women living alone or with nonrelatives.

Labor Force Participation

Although Americans are living longer, they are less likely than ever before to work during their later years. About three million older workers represent nearly 3 percent of the labor force. While the number of people over 65 has more than doubled since 1950, the number of workers over age 65 has remained steady. Due to a variety of factors, the participation rate in the labor force for older workers has declined markedly.

Ever since the establishment of the Social Security system half a century ago, Americans have considered age 65 the standard retirement age. In fact, the average age of retirement has been declining steadily, and today most Americans retire before age 65. In a 1978 Harris poll of retirees, two-thirds of the respondents had left work before age 65; the median age of retirement was 60.6 years.

For both sexes, participation in the labor force peaks in the 35- to 44-year-old age bracket and then declines with age, with the sharpest drop occurring during the early to mid-sixties (see Figure 1-16). In 1984, according to the Bureau of Labor Statistics, four in five men aged 55 to 59 were in the labor force, compared with one in four men aged 65 to 69 and one in nine men over age 70.

The proportion of older people in the work force has been dropping rapidly. Almost half of all men over 65 in 1950 were working, compared with only 16.3 percent today.

The pattern has been different for older women. During the last several decades, women have entered the work force in great numbers, largely counterbalancing the propensity of female workers to retire early. Labor force participation for women aged 55 to 64 rose from 27 to 42.7 percent. Participation among women over 65 declined slightly, edging downward from 10 percent in 1950 to 7.4 percent in 1987 (see Figure 1-17).

FIGURE 1-16 _____
Labor Force Participation by Age and Sex, 1987

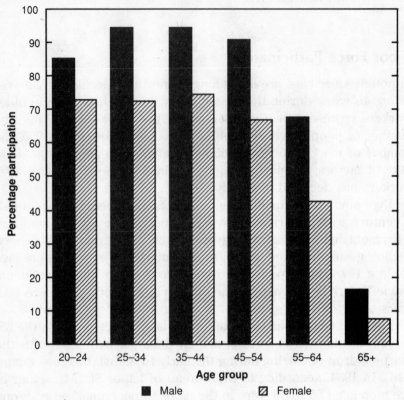

Source: Bureau of Labor Statistics, 1988

Factors Affecting Changes in Labor Force Participation

The downward trend in labor force participation among older people may be due to a variety of factors, including greater affluence, the enhancement of the Social Security system and private pension programs, mandatory retirement rules, and poor health.

Americans have enjoyed tremendous economic growth during this century, resulting in substantially higher real wages and income. Economist Victor Fuchs points out that for older men, this increased prosperity has raised the value of leisure (the "income effect" in economic theory) more than it has encouraged them to use their enhanced earning capacity to accumulate more money (the "price effect"). The reverse seems to be true for older women: higher real wages tend to increase labor force participation, perhaps because the income effect is dominated by the husband's (usually higher) income.

There is no question that the Social Security system has made retirement a more attractive option for many Americans, thus lowering the work force participation rate for older people. The value of Social Security benefits has been rising faster than wages; the gap in the rate of change widened during the 1970s. This provided continually increasing incentive for retirement. However, the current

FIGURE 1-17 _____
Labor Force Participation of Older Women, 1950–1987

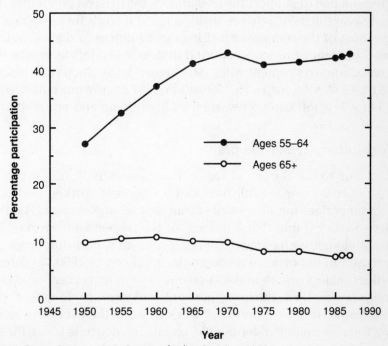

Source: Census Bureau, 1983; Bureau of Labor Statistics, 1988

rise in the ratio of older people in the work force seems to be tempering benefits growth relative to wage growth. *Nation's Business* magazine reports that during both 1982 and 1984 (the most recent year for which figures are available), wage increases exceeded benefit growth, the only such occurrences since at least 1950.

Another factor contributing to falling worker participation among older men is the declining incidence of self-employment. Older people who own their own businesses find it easier to modify their schedules without changing jobs or occupation. Conversely, wage- and salary-workers have less flexibility in their hours and wages. According to the Census Bureau, the proportion of self-employed workers plummeted during this century, as the American economy shifted from agriculture to industry and service. Not surprisingly, working men over 70 are over four times more likely to be farm workers than are all men over 25.

Mandatory retirement laws and age discrimination are often cited as reasons for older people leaving the work force. In fact, there is little evidence to support these claims. A 1981 Harris poll found that nearly two-thirds of retirees over 65 left the work force by choice, with most of the remainder retiring due to illness or disability. Less than 7 percent of retirees reported that they had left their jobs due to mandatory retirement rules (see Figure 1-18). Such rules will be even less of a factor in the future: in 1987 they were outlawed in all but a few job categories, such as firefighters and airline pilots.

Work among Older People

According to the Bureau of Labor Statistics, in 1987, 5.7 percent of those over 65 worked full time and 5.4 percent worked part-time. Retirement does not necessarily mean lack of employment. The 1981 Harris survey found that 5 percent of the respondents worked full time, and another 8 percent held part-time jobs. Part-time work has increased in importance among older workers. In 1960, 30 percent of older male workers and 43 percent of female workers held part-time jobs; by 1984, those proportions had risen to 46 and 61 percent, respectively. Yet part-time work remains the exception rather than the rule among older people, and its incidence is lower for single older people and very old people.

FIGURE 1-18 _____
Reasons for Retirement among Persons 65 and Older, 1981

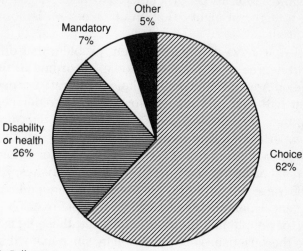

Source: Harris Poll, 1981

Thus, older people who do work are likely to spend under 40 hours per week at their jobs. Much of the flexibility to work part-time is due to the fact that over one-fourth of workers over 65 are self-employed (compared with only 9 percent of younger workers). While self-employment for the total population has dropped drastically during this century, the proportion of older people who work for themselves has grown steadily in recent years.

Labor force trends for older people have mirrored shifts in the American economy. Currently, both men and women over age 65 are most likely to be employed in the service sector, according to the Office of Technology Assessment (OTA). The Senate Committee on Aging reports that nearly three-fourths of workers over 65 hold white-collar jobs that do not involve physically taxing or dangerous tasks, often enabling workers to remain in the work force if they wish.

Older workers are more likely than younger workers to be employed by small businesses. The rapid increase in jobs within the small business sector may continue to provide employment opportunities for older people wishing to remain in the labor force.

Overall, then, a typical older worker is likely to be a white male working part-time at a white-collar job. He is likely to be under age 75 and in the labor force by choice. However, it is even more likely—by a factor of eight—that an older person is not in the labor force at all.

Older people have an unemployment problem that differs both in kind and degree from younger people, according to the Senate Committee on Aging. While the unemployment rate for people over 65 is about half that of younger workers, once older people lose their jobs, they tend to stay unemployed longer than do younger workers, experience a larger earnings loss in subsequent jobs, and are more apt to cease looking for another job after being laid off.

In 1987, according to the Bureau of Labor Statistics, 78,000 people over 65 were out of work, resulting in an unemployment rate of 2.5 percent. Unemployment rates for people over 65 are lower than those of people just under 65. However, these figures tend to understate the seriousness of the problem, since many discouraged older workers simply withdraw from the labor market when they are unsuccessful in finding a job. The Senate Committee on Aging reports that adding the proportion of discouraged older workers to those who are officially unemployed would effectively double the unemployment rate for older workers.

The Bureau of Labor Statistics projects that in 1995 there will be three million people over 65 in the labor force, roughly the same number as today. However, since both the total work force and the number of older people will grow by that year, older workers' participation rates will drop further. Workers over 65 will account for just 2 percent of the labor force, and less than 9 percent of people over 65 will be working.

The declining percentage of older workers, coupled with the burgeoning numbers of older people, has profound implications for our society. The overall percentage of Americans in the work force is dropping rapidly. In the future, there will be fewer younger people, most of whom will be working, to support a greater number of older people, most of whom will not. In 1950, approximately 50 workers paid taxes for each Social Security beneficiary; today each recipient is supported by about 3.4 workers, and during the next century that ratio will drop to two to one.

One way to illustrate this trend is to make the rough assumption that all people age 18 to 64 work to support all those under age 18 and over age 65. The ratios of older people to workers and children to workers are known as *support ratios*. Figure 1-19 shows that the number of people over 65 per 100 people age 18 to 64 (the elderly support ratio) will continue to rise for the foreseeable future. At the same time, the support ratio for children under 18 will decline as America becomes an older nation. The increased burden of caring for dependent elderly will in part be offset by the decreas-

FIGURE 1-19
Ratios of Old and Young to Working-Age Population, 1900–2040

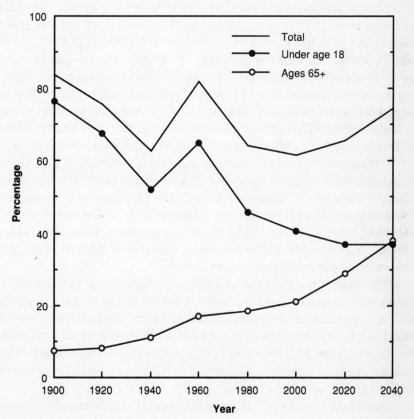

Source: Census Bureau, 1983

ing aggregate needs of younger people. However, most services for older people are publicly funded; in contrast, children are provided for largely by private (i.e., family) sources. This implies that the aging of America will demand either an increased tax base to finance care for older people, a privatization of services for older people, or some combination of the two.

Education

Today's older people are significantly less educated than the rest of the adult population. The average person over age 65 has 2.6 fewer years of formal education than the average person over 25.

As of 1982, one-third of all people between 65 and 74, and half of those over age 75, never went beyond elementary school, compared with less than one-sixth of the entire adult population over age 25. Less than half (44 percent) of people over 65—and only a third (35.3 percent) of those over age 75—had finished high school, while nearly three-fourths (71 percent) of all adults over age 25 had reached that level. Under 10 percent of people over 65 completed college versus 17.7 percent of the entire adult population. Figure 1-20 illustrates the differences in educational levels by age group.

Overall, women over 65 have completed an average of 11.1 years of school, slightly more than the 10.8 median years that men over 65 have completed. A greater proportion of older men graduated from college (10 percent versus 7 percent), but older men also are less likely than older women to have completed at least eight years of school. Thus, older men are overrepresented at both the high and low ends of the educational spectrum.

The educational gap between old and young, as measured by median years in school, has been narrowing for the past three decades and is expected to close during the next 10 years. Between 1970 and 1983, the median educational level for people over 65 rose from 8.7 to 11.0 years. By 1990, that figure is expected to increase to 11.9 years of school completed, compared with the current median of 12.6 years for all adults over 25.

Implicit in Figure 1-20 is the likelihood that this trend will continue, partly due to American immigration history and to the opportunities for World War II veterans created by the G.I. Bill. Immigrants comprise a far higher proportion of today's older population than do younger age groups; foreign-born older people have completed fewer years of school and suffer higher rates of illiteracy than those born in this country. The G.I. Bill enhanced educational opportunities for millions of Americans now in their sixties. All of these factors are likely to raise the average level of education among older people to near that of the rest of the adult population.

FIGURE 1-20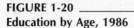
Education by Age, 1986

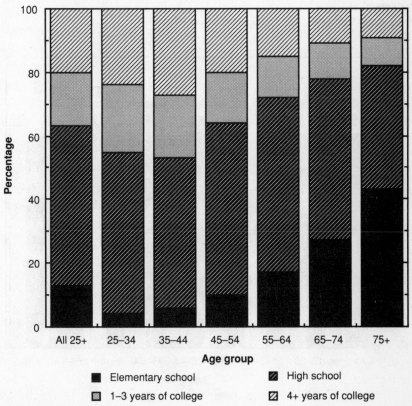

Source: Census Bureau, 1987

Voting Behavior

Older Americans are more likely than younger people to vote. The most complete voter information comes from the national elections in 1980 and 1984. Census data from those years show voter participation increasing up until age 65 or 70. Of all age groups, the highest voter participation rates in the 1984 election were found among voters 55 to 64 (72.1 percent) and those 65 to 74 (71.8 percent). People over 75 had a 61.2 percent voting rate in 1984. That year, the national rate of voter participation for all adults over 25 was only 59.9 percent (see Figure 1-21).

Among older people, white men are the most likely subgroup

FIGURE 1-21
Percentage Voting by Age Group, 1980 and 1984

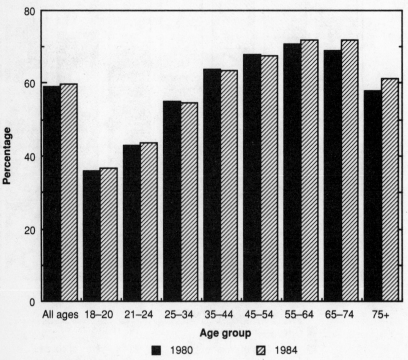

Source: Census Bureau, 1986

to vote, followed by white women, black men, and black women. Of those older Americans registered to vote but not voting in 1980, 40 percent reported illness as the cause.

Life Satisfaction Correlates

A variety of surveys have found an overwhelming majority of older people to be satisfied or very satisfied with their lives. About half of all older people place themselves in the highest response category offered. This may result partly from satisfaction being measured against expectations, which are colored by exaggerated negative images of aging. Presumably, many older people who are less happy with their lives are those living in institutions, who are generally excluded from opinion surveys.

FIGURE 1-22
Relative Contributions to Life Satisfaction among Elderly Persons

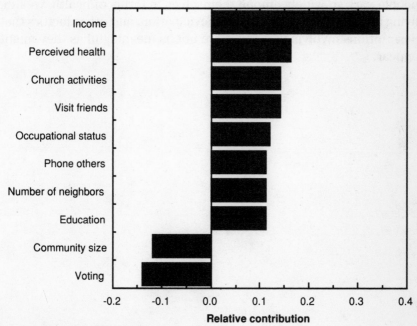

Source: Edmonds and Klemmeck, 1973

One major study attempted to determine factors important to life satisfaction for older people. Figure 1-22 (p. 53) illustrates the primary correlates found through the research. Note that income is by far the most significant factor, followed by perceived health status and a variety of issues involving participation in social activities. Note also that community size is inversely related to life satisfaction; that is, older people living in smaller towns—or in smaller communities within more populous areas—tend to be more satisfied with their lives.

The surprisingly high average degree of life satisfaction among older people underscores two characteristics of the socioeconomic status of older people. First, Americans of all ages tend to have unrealistically negative views of aging and older people that are not representative of the majority of the older population. The view of the typical older person as poor, lonely, and ailing simply is not supported by facts. Second, because the over-65 age group is the most diverse of all, accurate generalizations about socioeconomic or demographic characteristics are particularly difficult to make. Older people vary so widely among themselves in terms of health, wealth, living arrangements, labor force participation, and other factors that descriptions involving averages are not as meaningful as they might appear.

2

Understanding
and Marketing Eldercare

A number of well-publicized studies have made clear that older adults have greater health care needs than do younger people. Not only does the older population have *greater* health care needs, it also has *different* health care needs. While younger people's health care needs center around episodic care, the elderly's health care needs generally are chronic in nature.

Younger persons typically suffer from acute, episodic ailments: health problems that arise suddenly, can be treated as isolated conditions, and usually disappear within a reasonable period of time. The current medical system is designed to treat and care for the accidents and infectious diseases of youth.

In contrast, older adults tend to suffer from *chronic* diseases. In fact, 83 percent of the older population suffers from at least one such condition. This is not true for acute ailments: data from the National Center for Health Statistics show that older adults report less than half the rate of acute problems compared to the under-65 population. Arthritis, hypertension, diabetes, and other chronic ailments do not arise suddenly and rarely disappear. Additionally, older adults tend to suffer from *ambiplexy* (ambiguous, complex, multiple, interactive illness), which makes it inappropriate to isolate and treat each health problem separately.

The Current System
of Care for Older Adults

Health care needs for the older portion of the population fall into three major categories:

- *Acute medical needs.* The most obvious of elder health needs, these are served largely through physicians, registered nurses, and hospitals.

- *Ongoing health needs.* Given the prevalence of chronic disease and ambiplexy among the older population, infirm elders tend to require nonacute, often ongoing care. This can be delivered in an institution, in the home, or in the community, usually by any of a variety of health paraprofessionals.

- *Social support needs.* The complex and interactive nature of many elder health problems often requires coordination, information, family counseling, spiritual guidance, and other support functions. These are typically provided by nonmedical professionals, such as social workers, psychologists, care managers, clergy, or others.

Since the introduction of Medicare and its acute care orientation, the acute medical needs of older adults have been relatively well funded. Long-term care has fared worse, with Medicaid picking up the tab for nursing home care only when the recipient is impoverished. This underfunding has led to system-wide undercapacity, evidenced by the 95-plus percent occupancy rate in the nation's nursing homes. Social services have been funded most poorly of all, leading to a severe lack of availability of these services in most communities.

The American health care system today finds itself in a situation where the needs of its older citizen are not matched by the services available to them. First, the three major categories of health needs are addressed by three systems that are utterly separate in their structure and funding sources. Since many elders have a constellation of needs that involve all three categories, the separation of systems that serve those needs makes little sense in terms of quality of or access to care.

Second, the profound acute care bias of health care financing has resulted in an overdeveloped medical care system while stunting the growth and quality of long-term and social support services. These characteristics are the result of a health care system designed largely to serve the acute medical ailments of a youthful nation. Instead of redesigning our system to meet the needs of older adults, we continue to try to serve those needs through our acute care oriented medical system.

While touted as having the best health care system in the world, it is easy to find myriad examples in the United States that illustrate how we miss treating older adults appropriately. Here are just a few:

- *Medical training.* Our physicians have not been specially trained for the age wave. The National Institute on Aging recently estimated that fewer than 500 of the 550,000 doctors in America have completed fellowships in geriatric medicine. Although most physicians are quite able to effectively diagnose and treat most ailments associated with older adults, there are some areas in which training deficiencies are all too evident. For example, studies show that between 15 and 50 percent of all diagnosed cases of *irreversible* senile dementia are in fact *reversible*, yet the incorrect diagnosis typically leads to a lack of effort to reverse the condition.

- *Pharmaceuticals.* For all the positive effect drugs have on the health of older Americans, our pharmaceuticals do not always serve their purposes well. Most of the drugs used by older adults have not been tested on older adults, largely due to the difficulty of assessing the effect of a new drug on a metabolism already receiving several other medications. Yet this same polypharmaceutical research bugaboo creates a severe medical problem. Several studies have found that up to an astonishing 25 percent of hospital admissions for the over-65 population are related to adverse drug reactions or interactions.

- *Institutionalization.* We often institutionalize older persons to the detriment of their health and public funds because our delivery and financing systems have no suitable alternatives. A survey conducted for the National Center for Health Statistics found that barely a third of all nursing home residents are institutionalized because of the medical conditions listed on their admission records. The other two-thirds reside in nursing homes—at an average cost of about $60 per day—largely because adequate support is not available to keep them in the community or because no funding is available for such support.

Despite the hundreds of billions of dollars that we are spending on the health care of older Americans, the system we have created is inadequate and in many ways ineffective. But the age wave is making itself felt. The 63 million Americans over age 50, and the 76 million baby boomers who are starting to watch their parents age, represent a majority of Americans that is becoming increasingly dissatisfied with both the narrow focus and the cost of the current system. This population mass represents a political juggernaut that is already causing the emergence of a new health care system that will revolutionize the way the older adults receive care.

The Emerging Eldercare System

The discrepancy between the needs of our aging population and the structure of the American medical system is producing a new form of health care for our older population. This new structure, *eldercare*, is more than long-term care, and it is more than simply the superimposition of the acute medical care system designed for the young onto an older population. Eldercare is a system of medical, health, support, and life-style services designed to meet older adults' integrated needs. Eldercare recognizes that many of the older population's health needs do not involve medical care. Table 2-1 delineates the major differences between the acute medical care system and the emerging eldercare system.

The nature of eldercare may be diagrammed as in Figure 2-1. At the center is medical care, which serves the most life-threatening need and the one requiring the most expensive and intensive level

TABLE 2-1
Current Care versus Emerging Eldercare System

Current acute care system

Focuses on acute disease

Looks at isolated problems

Care delivered primarily in institutions

Care delivered primarily by physicians

Emerging eldercare system

Covers acute, chronic, support, and life-style needs

Looks at constellation of problems

Care delivered primarily in the community and the home

Care delivered by a range of professionals, paraprofessionals, and volunteers

---

of attention. The next ring involves health, including education and information, health promotion, nutrition, fitness, and similar issues. These services usually do not require the intervention of medically trained professionals. These two inner rings of the diagram represent what has typically been considered the health care system for older adults.

Moving outward from the center, however, there are two other rings that also are aspects of eldercare. One includes support services, such as transportation, care management, and chore and meal services. These activities do not provide direct medical or health services, but rather facilitate access to these or allow elders to function independently. The outermost ring, life-style, includes many of the daily activities of older adults, such as shopping, social events, financial management, and leisure travel. While not traditionally considered related to health, these needs in an aging nation are increasingly integrated with health needs, at least in the minds of the market. Health care providers who have recognized and acted upon the relevance of life-style to elder health concerns have been rewarded for their efforts.

FIGURE 2-1 _____
The Nature of Eldercare

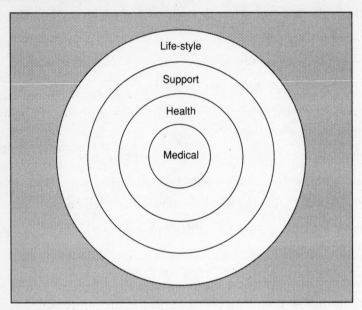

Source: Age Wave, Inc.

    The future eldercare system will be structured and reimbursed differently than the current system. Eldercare is a merger of the acute care, long-term care, and social service systems. Combining the capabilities of these systems is the only way to address the broad and integrated health and life-style needs of many older adults.

    There are three fundamental aspects of the eldercare system that must be recognized. First, eldercare recognizes and addresses the broad range of services that can meet the gamut of health, support, and life-style needs of older Americans. Through eldercare systems, the current gaps in health care and social systems are being filled in some communities. Second, in an eldercare system, the service delivery system is not concentrated solely on medical institutions, but is spread throughout the community at sites intended for the convenience of the *user* rather than the *provider*. Third, the variety of elder needs and the diversity and sheer number of providers necessitate a strong care management capability that the consumer can access through a single contact. This is known as a "one-stop shop" capability, and it is both absolutely crucial for and tremendously popular with older adults.

Thus, the emerging eldercare system offers a diversified continuum of services, arranged in a community-wide network, driven by a one-stop shop care-management system. The coordination capability is at the hub of the system, as illustrated in Figure 2-2. The hub controls utilization and serves as a doorway to the system. All providers are connected to one another via formal or informal relationships through the hub.

This change in the delivery system of health care will be paralleled by a shift in the financing of health care. The traditional fee-for-service system is losing ground to prepayment and capitation arrangements. Some experts predict that cost-based reimbursement will decrease to 5 percent of health care expenditures within three years. In addition to the rise of capitation and prepayment, Medi-

FIGURE 2-2 _____
The Eldercare Hub

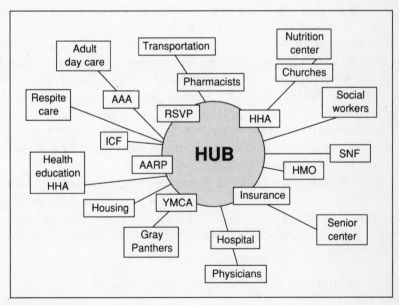

Source: Age Wave, Inc.

care and insurance copayments and deductibles are increasing. The emerging eldercare system will ultimately be financed on a prepaid, capitated basis, with direct payments from consumers accounting for an increasing share of total expenditures. Under this system, the organization filling the role of the hub in each network will be paid a predetermined amount to provide the majority of health and lifestyle needs to its members. With this system in place, the incentive to health care managers will be to place patients in the least intense, but most medically and socially appropriate, care level in order to minimize costs.

Eldercare Marketing Strategies

Successful providers of eldercare are recognizing the need for a new comprehensive array of services and are marketing these services to older adults, their caregivers, physicians, case managers, and local aging network. Although the marketing of eldercare is a new, specialized field, it draws on basic marketing principles. An understanding of the various target markets and their wants and needs is critical to success. Once a thorough understanding of the market and its components is in hand, the eldercare provider can begin addressing these needs. Marketing eldercare is an iterative process in which the market and the provider are in continual dialog: the eldercare provider designs and offers a service, the market responds, and the provider adjusts the service according to the market feedback and the provider's internal capabilities. No market is static, but the eldercare market in its early stages is particularly changeable. Successful eldercare marketers will be sensitive and responsive to these changing needs.

Once an eldercare provider has developed a strategic plan and eldercare services have been initiated, a marketing plan must be developed to make various hospital constituencies aware of and attracted to the program. The marketing process consists of three basic elements:

1. research into consumer needs and preferences,

2. development of a strategic marketing plan, and

3. devising and implementing a marketing program that includes both marketing communication tactics and other access channels.

These tasks differ for eldercare services as compared with those aimed at younger persons. Both market research and marketing communication are complicated by an extremely diverse population that generally cannot be measured or reached in concentrated settings, unlike younger age groups that typically can be accessed through schools or employers. The elderly have unique perceptual, cognitive, social, and psychological needs and preferences. Marketing strategy for eldercare must reflect these factors, as well as the large financial role of third-party payers and the important decision-making influence of families and physicians on older adults.

The Process of Marketing Health Care

At one time, marketing experts drew distinctions between marketing goods and services. The differences between distribution channels, communication channels, and audiences were thought to necessitate different marketing strategies. Today, as the lines between products and services themselves have blurred, a more sophisticated approach to marketing recognizes that a fundamental process must be understood and followed to market either goods or services. In health care, where the saleable items run the gamut from tangible goods such as durable medical equipment to pure services such as case management, the basic marketing process needs to be understood and followed in order to reach the appropriate markets and sell into these competitive markets.

Marketing is the effective creation and delivery of goods and services to a market willing to consume them at the going price. The key is the fit of the products with the preferences of the market. That requires both an understanding of the target population and a willingness to develop goods and services that meet its needs. Once these requirements are met, it is an easier task to communicate the benefits and availability of the products to a market desiring to buy them. Thus, the marketing process has three major components:

1. analyzing the market to determine its needs and wants,

2. creating or modifying goods and services to meet those needs, and

3. facilitating the awareness and use of the goods and services.

These three steps are listed in the order they should be taken and also in the order of decreasing difficulty for most businesses to accomplish.

Most organizations tend to put more focus on marketing communications than on solid market research and product development. Not surprisingly, they tend to be more successful at the communications tasks. There are many examples. The American auto industry has frequently demonstrated that it is better at promoting its products than at designing them to meet market needs. Both the computer and magazine industries have created marvelous products that no one wanted to buy. In these instances, companies have failed to recognize that effective marketing strategy is 80-percent empathy (understanding) and 20-percent creativity (design and communications).

When the health care industry began to take marketing seriously—in the early 1980s—executives rushed to embrace the third component, marketing communications. Many early attempts at marketing failed, or enjoyed only short-lived success, because they were nothing more than flashy advertising. Often the promotional campaigns were initiated with little or no serious market research. Consumers were bombarded with messages about the high quality of this hospital or the caring attitude of that health maintenance organization (HMO), with no reference to the many other attributes that consumers seek in health care providers.

Learning from their own and others' mistakes, many health care providers began to understand the critical nature of solid market research. While this aided them in understanding their markets, it still left them unclear as to how to differentiate their services from those of their competitors. This situation has remained, because health care organizations tend to have the most difficulty with the second component of marketing: creating new services or redefining existing ones to meet the needs and preferences of the marketplace.

Health care today remains far from being a market-driven industry. The good news is that organizations progressive enough to respond to market needs are garnering grateful consumers and generating widespread community support.

Marketing Basics: The Four Ps

Marketing theory states that any purchase decision involves four major elements in the minds of prospective consumers. Commonly known as *the four Ps*, they are product, price, place, and promotion.

The *product* is the good or service being offered. Prospective consumers view a product in terms of perceived value, which may differ from actual value. In health care, the difference between actual and perceived value may be great, due to the layperson's difficulty in judging the quality of a physician's skills or a hospital's equipment. Because health care holds such great personal importance for individuals, it is often difficult to assign a dollar value to it. For this reason, and because of the prevalence of third-party reimbursement, there is less sensitivity to the price of health care than to most other goods.

Place refers to the location at which the product can be purchased as well as the distribution channels through which it can be accessed. Often purchases can be increased simply by making the product more accessible. The place of health care use traditionally has been the hospital, nursing home, or physician's office. But this is changing. Much eldercare delivery is moving out of institutions into the community and the home. Some eldercare services, such as information, are delivered over telephone lines.

Price is the value that must be exchanged by the consumer to receive the product. Price is typically a dollar figure, but, in cases of exchanges, barters, or add-ons, price may be measured in some other currency. In health care, it is especially important to determine from whose perspective price is being considered. For example, a $5000 hospital stay for a 70-year-old man might be paid for by a combination of Medicare, private insurance, and out-of-pocket funds. The going price of the service will differ for each payer; perhaps Medicare will pay $4000, private insurance $800, and the individual $200.

The fourth P, *promotion*, refers to the ways in which potential purchasers are made aware of and encouraged to buy the product. Marketing communications—notably advertising—comes to mind first. But promotion has many other elements, including such things as price discounts, bonuses, and add-ons. Some promotions involve offering a perceived value to prospective consumers in exchange for simply making the effort to try a product.

Unique Aspects of Health Care Marketing

While the fundamentals of marketing must be observed in marketing health care, as they are in marketing other goods and services, there are a number of important differences that cannot be overlooked.

To begin with, marketing has not always been a component of the health care industry. Until recently, health care was a provider-driven industry, and buyers (third-party payers and individuals) had little say in what services were provided and how they were delivered. But the cost-containment imperative and the increase in health care consumerism recently have combined to bring market forces to bear on the industry. Still, health care remains somewhat buffered from the full force of the marketplace.

Second, ethical issues take on special significance in health care marketing. Ethically, there is a marked difference in persuading a consumer to trade in a relatively new car for an upscaled model and in leading a patient to consider surgery that may be unnecessary. Although little health care marketing has reached so crass a level, the potential exists for abuse.

Third, health care marketing is unique because the consumer is not always the purchaser. In most fields, the purchase decision-maker, the payer, and the user are all the same individual or organization. In health care, a physician might decide (effectively) to purchase a pharmaceutical that will be paid for by Blue Cross and used by a patient. Thus, health care marketing efforts often must be directed at multiple audiences.

Finally, because health care is so important to individuals and to society, its value goes beyond that of most other products. The mission of most health care providers is to serve their communities, rather than merely to earn profits. Therefore, good health care marketing may result in the creation and enhanced utilization of some unprofitable services or possibly the avoidance of services that might be profitable but not beneficial to health. In short, the purpose of marketing in health care encompasses both health enhancement and business gain.

More Marketing Basics: The Five Steps

Again, marketing theory offers a series of fundamental steps to successful marketing. The marketing process consists of five distinct steps: market analysis, market planning, product planning, marketing tactics, and promotional strategy.

Market Analysis:
Consumers and Competitors

The first phase of marketing involves understanding what the market wants and how well those wants are currently being served. This begins with thorough market research into two areas:

- The needs and preferences of the population being surveyed

- Consumers' views on the products and services currently available

In addition, an audit of the sponsoring organization and its competitors should be done to determine:

- the overall perception (brand image) of each major provider, and

- the capabilities of each major provider.

Many obvious conclusions usually can be drawn immediately. For example, initial surveys may identify a strong need for a particular product or the oversupply of a service within a market segment. In any case, good analysis can generate additional insight. Analysis should endeavor to:

- detect patterns among market reactions to existing products and services;

- make sense of market needs and preferences in terms of the *potential* products and services that might be offered;

- determine not just *how* consumers feel about each provider, but *why;* and

- compare what the various providers offer, and which providers hold significant competitive advantages over the others.

A thorough market analysis, based on sound research, is the foundation for any marketing effort. Incomplete or faulty analysis makes the remainder of the process a hit-or-miss affair.

Market Planning: Selection and Segmentation

Once a thorough analysis of the market and all major players has been completed, an overall strategy must be developed. This begins with the selection of the market(s) to be addressed. Of course, the more broadly the market is defined, the larger the universe of potential buyers and the more difficult it is to tailor products and promotions for that population.

The first market selection issue is whether to address the older market at all. Most health care providers will choose to do so rather than risk losing the largest and fastest-growing pool of potential customers. The second issue—determining which portions of the older adult market to address—is often ignored.

Many providers decide to target the over-65 population, but lack a rationale for using that age cutoff. If their goal is simply to build market share, they might target the whole mature market (50-plus) or even the entire population. Medicare eligibility starts at age 65, but few providers prefer Medicare patients to private-pay ones.

Some providers construct elaborate market programs that attract low-income elders when none or few of the physicians on their medical staffs are willing to accept Medicare assignment. Others focus on the wealthy elderly despite their original mission to serve the poor. An overall strategy for market selection must be developed in concert with organizational goals. A marketing program should develop services for, and promote them to, the population groups that the provider wishes to serve.

Once the target market has been selected, it must be segmented into meaningful subdivisions. Market segmentation involves dividing the total market into identifiable groups whose members all share common characteristics. Segmentation is done for purposes of both effectiveness and efficiency. The more clearly the market is segmented, the easier it is to design and sell products that each segment will want to buy.

How should the older market be segmented? This, of course, depends on market selection and the broader organizational strategy. Since the ultimate goal of the segmentation process in eldercare is to better serve and/or better sell services to older adults, a good rule of thumb is to segment based on either health needs or purchasing behavior, or both. Thus, segmentation by age group (e.g., 65 to 74, 75 to 84, 85-plus) often is less helpful than segmentation by health status (e.g., presence of heart disease) or by influences on health care decisions (e.g., presence or absence of a regular physician).

Product Planning: Development or Redefinition

Market analysis and market selection should lead to product offerings that are responsive to the needs of the segments being targeted. New and/or existing products can be involved. Often this phase of the marketing process includes refining or modifying existing products.

Health care providers traditionally have offered products or services based on the availability of new medical procedures or technologies, rather than in response to market needs. As the industry becomes more market-driven (due to increasing demands by payers and consumers), this orientation will change. Successful providers already are conducting more market research and developing new services that are demanded by their local consumer base.

An eldercare product or service may need to appeal to multiple constituencies. These could include older adults, their families, physicians (both primary care and specialist), nurses, third-party payers (government and private), elder organizations, and a host of other possible entities. Thus, products must be designed with an eye to all parties that might be involved in the purchase decision. Traditionally, health care products have been created more to satisfy providers and payers than to meet consumer needs.

A new-product concept can be tested through surveys or focus groups. These types of research can help refine new ideas, reduce the possibility of failure, and suggest marketing communication strategies. Market testing helps ensure that the first P of marketing—*product*—will be responsive to the needs of potential customers.

Marketing Tactics: Pricing and Distribution

Once the market has been analyzed and segmented, and appropriate products and services have been created, several tactical marketing decisions must be made. One of these is *price*, the second P of marketing. It is important to keep in mind that prices are signals to the market: high-priced items are more likely to be perceived as being high quality than low-priced items, and vice versa.

In health care, prices have historically been based on estimated cost, plus a margin for profit. In recent years, third-party payers have tightened payment restrictions, often resulting in providers' receiving reimbursement that falls short of their costs. Increasingly, pricing in health care is effectively being set by the buyer—insurance companies, HMOs, and the government. Often prices must be set low for competitive reasons.

While some experts predict that the purchasing pendulum will swing back to reward quality, the continuing rapid growth in health care expenditures is likely to maintain the focus on price for some time.

Other important tactical decisions must be made regarding distribution channels. The success of a product may depend largely on how consumers can access it. An example is the local convenience store. Consumers do not shop there for price (which tends to be high) or quality (which often is low) or diversity of merchandise (which typically is limited). Rather, consumers shop there for ease of access; such stores usually are conveniently located, with express checkout lines and plenty of free parking.

Elements of access include—but go beyond—location, waiting time, and parking availability. Delivery speed, acceptance of personal checks or credit cards, proximity to other frequently visited sites (such as supermarkets or banks), hours of operation, and many other issues affect access.

Similarly, decisions about distribution channels can have enormous impact on the success of a product. Firms such as Mary Kay Cosmetics and Amway have done very well by selling and distributing through individuals rather than retail stores.

For health care providers, issues of access and distribution are changing. In the past, most care was delivered in physicians' offices, hospitals, and nursing homes. The widespread implementation of prospective payment plans in the 1980s has encouraged health care to move outside of institutional settings. The move toward an eldercare orientation will cause care to become even more community- and home-based.

Innovative eldercare providers are reaching out into their communities as much as possible. Some are opening aging resource centers in shopping malls to maximize traffic flow. Other providers are collaborating with senior centers, churches, YMCAs, or other community-based organizations to enhance access to health care. Another way to encourage use of services is to remove psychological or physical barriers to access; many providers offer transportation programs to allow elders who do not drive to use their services.

Promotional Strategy: Marketing Communications and Access Channels

Promotional strategy should be based solidly on research, market selection, product development, and pricing and distribution decisions. One aspect of promotion is marketing communications: advertising, brochures, telemarketing, press releases, public relations campaigns, and the like.

This area tends to be overemphasized in most marketing efforts. Many attractive and well-funded marketing communications campaigns fail because of insufficient market research, poor product development, bad strategy, overpricing, or any of a number of faulty marketing decisions.

A good marketing communications campaign begins with an understanding of the media habits and life-style patterns of the target population. Considerations of frequency, reach, and expense all should play heavily in a communications strategy. Campaigns may be oriented toward general image advertising or toward a specific product.

Promotion, the fourth P of marketing, goes beyond advertising. It includes techniques to enhance the likelihood of purchase, such as discounts and bonuses. It may include familiarizing potential consumers with a product, as with open houses or travel subsidies. An unusual example is the midwestern hospital that offered free rides from the local senior center to older adults who wanted to watch cataract surgery; after seeing and understanding the procedure, many spectators requested the operation for themselves!

Of course, promotion also includes direct sales efforts. Sales is a relative newcomer to health care, especially to hospitals. Many hospitals have created sales forces to sell services to corporations and other potential group buyers. Health maintenance organizations use salespersons (whose titles usually include the terms "marketing" or "professional relations") to communicate with individuals, employers, and providers.

A good promotional campaign includes a means to track its effectiveness. The nature of the evaluative mechanism depends on the purpose of the campaign. If advertising is directed at general image improvement, image surveys might be taken before and after the campaign and the results compared. If a promotional effort is aimed at direct product sales, success might be measured by a controlled experiment in which the effort is directed at one of two identical groups; if the study is carefully done, the difference in product sales can be attributed to the promotion. Such tracking efforts should gauge both effectiveness and efficiency, for example, the cost per thousand for reaching the target population.

Health care providers have been advertising heavily for the past several years. Hospital advertising budgets, for example, reached an average of $158,300 in 1987, according to *Hospitals* magazine. However, a lack of careful research into market needs, combined with an orientation toward promoting existing products rather than developing new, market-responsive offerings, has rendered many advertising campaigns ineffective. Of course, most health care providers do not know with any certainty just how well they have spent their advertising dollars, since few organizations have the means to track communications efforts.

Not all eldercare communications are directed at older adults. Some are geared toward their adult children, physicians, elder organizations, clergy, volunteers, donors, or others. Each target group must be researched carefully and approached differently.

Marketing Continues for the Life of the Product or Service

Although it is logical to consider the phases of marketing sequentially, the activities should overlap. Marketing is an ongoing process in which the last stage is also the first step of the next round.

For example, market research and analysis should be conducted at several points in the marketing process. Basic research should be used to determine the needs and wants of the population to be served. Product testing should follow the product development phase. Additional market testing can be helpful to refine a proposed marketing communications campaign. Finally, research can gauge the success of a marketing effort by testing for changes in attitudes toward the sponsoring organization.

Product planning also should be an ongoing process. Many ideas for new goods or services are likely to arise during or even before market analysis. Tactical decisions on pricing and distribution often lead to rethinking the original product to enhance the likelihood of its success. Feedback from a marketing communication campaign can lead to modification of existing products or the creation of new ones.

Initially an organization may develop an overall marketing strategy based on market analysis and then devise tactics to carry out that strategy. However, it is common, after some experience in a marketplace has been gained, for tactics to drive strategy. For example, a health care provider may decide to create a product aimed at a certain ethnic group living within a particular area, and price that product accordingly. However, the product might fail within that target market, but do rather well with a group that was originally outside of the target market. In that case, the experience might cause the provider to rethink tactics (so as to appeal to the original group) or strategy (to enhance success within the second group), or both.

Chapter 3, Eldercare Services, explores the development, implementation, and marketing of 23 eldercare services. In that chapter and Chapter 4, Eldercare Case Studies, the principles of designing and marketing actual programs are shown in practical settings. Once the theory of developing and marketing programs is well understood, additional insight can be gained by examining the operational details of existing programs. The hope is that by looking at real world examples, those providers beginning or refining their eldercare programs will not be forced to "reinvent the wheel."

Eldercare Services

3

Because older adults tend to have not one health problem, but rather a constellation of conditions, it is especially important to think about treating the person and not simply the disease at hand. In Chapter 2, Understanding and Marketing Eldercare, the concept of the eldercare infrastructure was discussed as a way to tie together and provide access to needed services. An eldercare program is more than the sum of its parts. The quality of a program is measured not only by the quality of its individual services but by its overall comprehensiveness.

We will now study 23 eldercare services individually. Although there is a risk to focusing on the "trees" when the "forest" is so important, there is also a benefit, from a business perspective, to analyzing each major service as a stand-alone operation.

The varied nature of eldercare services makes generalizations difficult. In addition, due to the rapidly changing nature of the field, little published information is available that explores the details of planning, marketing, and delivering the spectrum of eldercare services. This chapter, while not intended by itself to enable a health care manager to implement a program, examines the salient characteristics of a wide variety of services so that managers can decide which ideas to pursue further. Sources for further information are mentioned throughout the section.

Because many eldercare services are just emerging, reliable central data sources often are unavailable. The information in this chapter was gleaned from the authors' experience and from hundreds of site visits and interviews with hospital operating executives, elder service managers, community providers, industry organizations, academic experts, and health care consultants. Most general facts and figures are mentioned as rough guidelines and should not be used as a basis for planning. There is no substitute for research into local conditions and regulations.

Designing the Eldercare Environment

Older adults, due to changes in physical and mental condition and life-style needs and preferences, require programs and facilities that differ in many respects from those aimed at younger persons. Because America has been a youth-oriented society for so long, most of our systems and structures were designed to suit the needs of youth or middle-age. Chairs, doorknobs, and interior lighting are just a few examples of products designed for the young that are inadequate for many older persons. The duration of traffic signals and the size of commonly used typefaces are better suited to the ambulatory and perceptive capabilities of the young than the old.

Environmental Design for
Inpatient Facilities

The appropriateness of an environment is measured by its suitability to its inhabitants. Because there is wide variation among the elderly in terms of mobility, general health, perceptual faculties, and social preferences, no environment can be designed to meet the needs of all older persons. However, each level of eldercare should be housed in a facility designed for the characteristics of persons likely to need such care. Inpatient, personal, or long-term centers, as well as informational or educational programs, should include specific features to enhance their effectiveness in serving the elderly. Often these features are important enough to affect care quality significantly.

There are three primary issues that eldercare designers should consider when planning facilities for older adults:

- mobility limitations,

- perceptual changes, and

- patterns of social interaction.

Mobility Limitations: Some older adults, especially those likely to be found in and around health care facilities, may be restricted in their ability to move around. The degree of mobility limitation can range from mildly arthritic joints to the inability to move without assistance. Experts estimate that more than half of institutionalized residents in skilled and intermediate care facilities use wheelchairs and should be considered when designing an acute inpatient or long-term care facility, or any building or room that older adults are likely to use. Entry and exit ramps are helpful, but better still are facilities built on a level plane with no steps or inclines whatsoever. Floor moldings or depressions that might hinder an older person's wheelchair should be avoided or removed. Because many older adults have difficulty wheeling in tight circles, pathways connecting rooms and corridors should allow plenty of room for turning. Plans should not be based on standard wheelchair width, but should add 12 to 24 inches for elbow extension beyond wheel hubs.

In addition to wheelchair movement, well-designed eldercare facilities will consider the needs of older wheelers once they reach their destinations. Wheelchair footrests add nearly 12 inches between an occupant and a work surface, unless the surface is designed to allow footrests to extend beneath it. This problem also affects bathroom mirrors, storage closets, activity rooms, kitchens and other fixtures. A wheelchair generally is higher than a conventional seat, which makes the height of some tables and other surfaces inappropriate for wheelers. Many facilities frequented by older persons have well-furnished lounges or common areas that allow little space for wheelchairs, often leading to attractive but unused rooms.

Of course, not all mobility limitations involve wheelchairs. Many older adults are quite able to walk, but are less certain than younger persons of their footing and balance. Many hospitals, originally designed more to inhibit the spread of infectious diseases than to facilitate comfort for older patients, have smooth floors waxed to a high gloss to demonstrate cleanliness. Even floors specially treated to prevent slipping resemble ice-skating rinks to many older persons with deteriorating eyesight and poor balance. Many falls result from older adults shifting body weight inappropriately to avoid skidding on highly waxed, nontextured floors.

Floors should be carpeted for maximum safety. Many facilities have avoided carpeting areas used heavily by older adults due to concerns over incontinence. However, durable indoor-outdoor carpeting can withstand frequent cleanings and will reduce the risk of falls. If the floor is not carpeted, a wooden or other relatively rough surface is desirable. Most dangerous of all are throw rugs, which often lead to slipping or tripping and should be avoided.

Bathrooms must be designed with an eye to mobility limitations of older adults. Support bars on walls and in showers are important safety precautions. Mirrors that can be pulled out from the wall accommodate elders with failing eyesight. Bath mats are as dangerous as throw rugs and should be avoided. Care should be taken to keep the floor from becoming wet and slippery, perhaps by installing a drain in the center of the room or by carpeting the floor.

Perceptual Changes: Changes in all five senses typically accompany aging, even in a healthy individual. Sight and hearing have particular relevance for eldercare design, although the other senses also should be considered.

During the normal aging process, the eye's lens begins to yellow and thicken, creating an uneven lens surface. In addition, the muscles that contract and dilate the pupils become less responsive. These changes have dramatic implications for vision. The uneven thickening of the lens makes older persons extremely sensitive to glare, whether from bright lights, shiny floors, bathroom fixtures, metallic surfaces, or other sources. The yellowing of the lens increases the need for light: a typical 80-year-old requires about three times as much light as a 20-year-old. Sluggish pupil dilation and contraction increases the amount of time an older adult needs to adjust to a differently lit environment or to recover from a flash of light. Color perception also is affected by changes in the eye: light pastels, such as blues, beiges, and pinks, and darker shades, such as black, brown, and charcoal, are hard to distinguish in many settings.

Design and construction of eldercare facilities should address these changes in several ways. Lighting should be bright but diffuse, and bulbs or tubes should be shielded. Indirect lighting is best. If cost considerations dictate use of fluorescent lights—whose flickering is more evident to the old than to the young—cover the bulbs with a cove or valence, and make sure to maintain ballast adjustment. Ideally, incandescent bulbs of 40 to 60 watts should be used; test different wattages to see whether residents can read comfortably at various intensities.

Lighting for close-work tasks must be strong, and supplemental sources should be used when possible for reading, table games, and other focused activities. Mood lighting is ineffective for older adult settings. Many older persons look downward when they walk, and, therefore, light should be directed to their path. Nightlights in bedrooms should be avoided, because they create large and eerie shadows that can frighten a disoriented older person. It is better to leave the bathroom or hall light on with the door slightly ajar.

Glare can be reduced by using nonskid carpets and by covering tables and work surfaces with tablecloths. Windows frequently present glare problems if they are not tinted or cannot be shaded appropriately; using tinted glass, smaller panes, or louvered window shades that allow in natural light while blocking the direct rays of the sun help alleviate glare. Colors can be used to contrast figures and backgrounds, such as dark letters on light signs or pale furniture on a dark carpet. Supergraphics, large figures or symbols created for purposes of information or orientation, should not be so large or highly placed as to extend beyond an older person's range of vision.

Visual cues can be used to assist mentally or perceptually impaired elders in orienting themselves. Having distinctly different decoration in each hallway, for example, reduces confusion for those moving around a building. Rooms can be marked with nameplates using three-quarter-inch high letters of uniform height; ideally these letters should be recessed rather than raised to avoid shadowing. Some inpatients may prefer to fashion their own name plates, perhaps also including a photograph or other personal item.

Hearing, too, is affected by aging. An older adult has more difficulty than a younger person in distinguishing a sound or voice from a background of competing noises. This competition may involve conversation, traffic, background music, electrical hums, a heating or air-conditioning unit or some other ongoing source of noise. Background noise is especially distracting for older persons and may cause confusion or create tension. A well-designed eldercare facility will consider the sources of potentially distracting sounds and will minimize their exposure to older persons. Sound absorbing furnishings will reduce echoes and deaden background noise.

Another change in hearing that occurs with aging is the decreased ability to perceive high-frequency sounds. Unfortunately, staff personnel tend to raise their voices in pitch as well as volume when speaking to older persons, often raising the noise level without significantly enhancing communication. Similarly, older adults often will increase the volume on a television set until staff complain of headaches. Many public-address systems, as well as radio or television receivers, introduce proportionately more high frequency sounds as volume is increased. Eldercare facilities can alleviate these problems by acquiring the capability to differentially raise bass tones relative to the treble, perhaps by routing the television sound through an adjustable stereo amplifier. Some public-address systems have the same capability. In addition, common areas can be designed and furnished so that residents can sit close to one another and communicate without shouting.

Patterns of Social Interaction: Many hospitals and nursing homes were designed to facilitate interaction between patients and visitors or among residents. However, numerous architectural features and interior furnishings actually serve just the opposite function, while simultaneously decreasing the comfort level of all involved.

For example, many institutional hallways are long and unchanging, and are viewed by older persons with poor depth perception as caverns extending infinitely. Stripes or patterns along the floor intended to help guide residents to particular destinations can be distracting or confusing. Some floor patterns resemble steps. As noted above, shiny floors can appear unsafe. A handrail on the wall can improve the comfort level of older adults who walk unsteadily.

Equally important, residents must have a place they wish to go if they are to leave their rooms. Lounges often are underutilized due to inappropriate design. Flickering fluorescent lights or glare from large windows can be distracting, and acoustical factors often cause annoying background noise. Furnishings frequently are poorly conceived, usually consisting of vinyl couches or linked chairs. Older persons need individual chairs so that they can move closer to others to hear them more comfortably, or simply to have the option of gathering in social groupings of various sizes. Ample space should be left for wheelchairs.

Unfortunately, most furniture specifically designed for older adults is inappropriate for them. Low, soft couches may be comfortable to sit in but are difficult to rise from. Although vinyl seats are easily cleaned after use by incontinent patients, that is no reason for entire chairs or couches to be covered with vinyl. Such furniture often is uncomfortable and usually is unattractive. Rocking chairs are dangerous and may tip over. A far better alternative is a platform rocker, built like a stationary swing, which is safe and comfortable and provides good exercise.

Pedestal tables, which are popular in eldercare facilities because they have no outside legs to interfere with wheelchairs, are in fact very dangerous: older persons often brace themselves against the outside of the table when rising and tip both the table and themselves. All tables should have four sturdy legs. Chairs should have arms that extend forward beyond the seats to aid in rising. Overall, furniture should be functional and varied to reflect the diverse mobility needs and preferences of older adults.

Many eldercare facilities have limited options for moderately sized gatherings. Most acute care hospitals or long-term care facilities provide opportunities for patients or residents to interact with one or two other persons (in the bedrooms) or with a large crowd (in the lounges), but few areas are suitable for family-size groups.

Socialization can be enhanced by offering a call system near activity centers, so that residents feel comfortable leaving their rooms. The availability of a bathroom and drinking water will increase the time that residents will stay in common areas. For inpatient hospital units that primarily serve older adults, rooms with three or four beds often are used to promote socialization. For example, Durham County General Hospital, in North Carolina, has a four-bed room on its geriatric inpatient unit in order to stimulate social and mental activity.

Considerations for
Outpatient and Community-Based Programs

Many of the issues discussed above are relevant to outpatient or community-based programs. An aging resource center must be accessible to the frail elderly. A health education program should be designed with aging-related perceptual changes in mind, regardless of the particular media used. Health fairs must be held in buildings with doors that are light enough to be opened by an older person, preferably with door levers rather than knobs.

Information Sources

There are many considerations to weigh in designing facilities and programs for the elderly. Planners should seek input from persons with a history of success in eldercare design. However, since the majority of health care facilities are inappropriate for older adults in some respects, experience may not be enough. One potential source of advice for inpatient facility design is the local foundation for the blind, which is accustomed to addressing issues of access and orientation for disabled persons.

Phoenix Memorial Hospital, is also a good source of information about designing facilities for the elderly. Phoenix Memorial Hospital has designed and constructed a 24-bed inpatient skilled nursing unit especially for older adults. Contact Phoenix Memorial Hospital at P.O. Box 21207, Phoenix, AZ 85036; (602) 238-3401.

Another excellent resource is Lorraine G. Hiatt, Ph.D., a New York-based environmental consultant with experience in facility design for the elderly and disabled. Contact her at 200 West 79th Street, 7N, New York, NY 10024; (212) 874-7713.

Adult Day Care

Adult day care involves services provided in a variety of settings, including hospitals, nursing homes, congregate housing, and religious and community centers, as well as through home health care and homemaker programs. Services are provided on weekdays, usually between 7 AM and 5:30 PM, to individuals who return home in the evening. Adult day care allows older adults who cannot function completely independently to remain in their community and to avoid or delay institutionalization. Services provided may include skilled nursing care; physical, occupational, and speech therapy; social, nutritional, and recreational services; and transportation.

There are three general types of adult day care programs. *Medical day care* emphasizes health needs of participants and arranges for therapeutic services recommended by a physician. *Maintenance programs* focus on both physical and psychological needs of clients, and generally are longer in duration than medical programs. *Social day care* is less medically oriented and may emphasize health maintenance or social activities. Many adult day care programs provide a mix of medical, maintenance, and social services. Adult day care may also be called day health care, medical day care, day treatment, or geriatric day care. However, adult day care usually is distinguished from day hospital care, which emphasizes intensive rehabilitation in a hospital setting without the costs of room and board.

The National Institute for Adult Daycare (NIAD) reports that there are approximately 1700 adult day care programs nationwide, up from 1200 as recently as 1985. This does not represent steady growth, but a great many new programs opening even as others close. Only about 10 percent are for-profit programs. Only about 5 percent are hospital-based, but that proportion is growing rapidly. Most such programs are located in separate facilities outside of the sponsoring institutions. Hospital-based programs tend to be more medically oriented than independent adult day care centers.

One specialized type of adult day care involves dementia patients. A growing number of hospitals are offering Alzheimer's day care, which involves a mix of maintenance and social care. Although such programs must address special concerns, most of the management issues are similar to those of general adult day care centers, which usually serve many dementia patients.

The federal government has not established any regulations for adult day care, but 41 states and the District of Columbia require certification for funding.

Value: Adult day care benefits functionally impaired elderly patients by providing enough support to allow them to remain in the community, thus preventing unnecessary or premature placement in a hospital or nursing home. Most individuals prefer a community-based care program to an institution. Adult day care also offers an opportunity to socialize with peers outside of the home and provides a broad spectrum of services in a single setting. The client's family benefits by having regular and reliable respite care and by receiving counseling from professionals experienced in the challenges of caring for the chronically ill.

Hospitals reap several benefits from offering adult day care services. Such a program facilitates the discharge of patients and enhances their continuity of care. From a marketing perspective, adult day care retains discharged inpatients within the hospital system, draws new clients from the community, promotes the institution to the patient's family members, and provides a visible indication of the hospital's commitment to serving older adults. Additionally, adult day care complements other hospital programs, such as home care and rehabilitation, thus providing an important element in the broad continuum of services that will define the eldercare system of the future.

Cost: Capital costs for an adult day care program vary greatly, depending on the need for facility construction or renovation. Programs operated within a hospital or community center may need little initial investment, since minimum space requirements include an accessible large room and toilet facilities. Most centers require some renovation, primarily for accessibility of the room(s), toilets, and parking.

A typical maintenance-oriented adult day care program with a 30-person capacity might require start-up costs of $7500 for office equipment, $2500 for medical equipment, and perhaps $2500 more for additional supplies. Kitchen equipment will add $3000 to $4000 if the program is cooking rather than purchasing its meals.

Operating costs vary with staff size, which in turn depends in part on program orientation. The American Hospital Association (AHA) reports estimated per diem costs ranging from $15 to $45 per participant. The NIAD estimates average daily costs at $27 to $31 per participant, exclusive of transportation. Annual operating budgets may range from $50,000 to $200,000, depending on program size and orientation. A greater emphasis on medical services increases total costs. Staffing is the largest expense; food usually is second.

Transportation costs average about $5 per day per participant. On the average, 42 percent of the participants will have their own transportation, but this figure will vary tremendously between sites. Purchase and operation of one van can require $40,000 for the first year. However, some of this cost can be defrayed by sharing the van with other programs. The scheduling requirements of adult day care dovetail with those of a meals-on-wheels service, which typically delivers meals at lunchtime. Additionally, a local business may donate used vans or serve as a partial or total sponsor in return for having its name displayed prominently on the vehicle.

State licensing regulations often require the presence of certain professionals, such as nurses and physical therapists. This affects program costs, which are largely staff-related and, therefore, tend to be fixed. However, revenues are attendance-related and, thus, are variable. Typically, only 30 to 60 percent of enrolled clients will attend on any given day. Thus, program attendance levels are critical to average daily per-client costs.

Staffing: While no widely accepted standards exist for adult day care program staffing, many states have minimum requirements for certified programs. Program size and orientation also affect staffing needs. So do hours: only about half of all programs nationwide are open for an eight-hour day. All programs have an administrator who typically has a background in nursing, social work, gerontology, or public health. Core staff includes nurses, social workers, and recreational therapists. Medically oriented adult day care programs also have licensed physical and occupational therapists.

Although physicians generally are not on the staff of adult day care programs, they often are involved in developing personal care plans for patients. Other staff may include nursing and dietary aides, activity helpers, clerical staff, and one or more drivers. Volunteers and interns can supplement staff and provide an excellent means to expand services without significantly increasing costs.

A typical adult day care program might be staffed by a full-time registered nurse (RN) with geriatric training, a social worker, a recreational therapist, and a nursing aide (or several part-time aides). In addition, the program administrator and secretary may be either part-time or full-time workers. A part-time driver or driver/custodian would round out the staff. While staff-to-participant ratios vary by program, NIAD reports that most adult day care services have between five and eight participants for each staff member.

A recent national survey of adult day care centers, performed by the Oklahoma Department of Human Services and the Department of Family Medicine at Oklahoma University, found that the average program employed 8.3 full-time equivalent (FTE) paid staff members and had 7 FTE volunteers. Paid full-time employees average 37.2 hours per week of work, part-time employees 19.0 hours, and volunteers 10.7 hours. These figures were for nearly 100 programs with average enrollments of 52 and daily attendance averaging 28.

Revenues: Adult day care programs are funded by a variety of public, private, and philanthropic sources. No single revenue source covers all services included in a comprehensive program. The difficulty of funding seems to be increasing even as adult day care is becoming more popular. This is partly because the intensity of care has risen. According to a 1987 Institute for Health and Aging study of the impact of changes in Medicare diagnosis-related group (DRG) policies since 1984, adult day care programs have reported increased revenues from first-party payers, Medicaid and private insurance, while the participants required more hours of care, heavier supervision, and had more severe functional impairments. Costs of adult day care programs generally exceed revenues by a considerable amount, and most hospital-based programs are subsidized by the sponsoring institution or its associated foundation.

Medicare does not recognize adult day care as a reimbursable service, but may pay for skilled nursing and rehabilitation, physical, occupational, and speech therapy through Part B. When such reimbursement is available, Medicare pays an average of about $20 per day. Medicaid is a more prominent payer: adult day care is an optional service under Medicaid, and several states offer reimbursement—not necessarily enough to cover costs—through their programs. Some states fund adult day care through the 2176 waiver program. And Congress has been considering legislation that would provide federal funding for adult day care as an option in the provision of long-term care.

Social service block grants (SSBGs), formerly Title XX, are another source of program funds. Because states have discretion over the proportion of SSBG funds to be spent on adult day care, the amount of funding varies widely. Social services, such as meals, transportation, client needs assessment, and social therapy, are more often reimbursed by SSBGs than are health services. Many states also use funds from Title III-B of the Older Americans Act to pay for meals, transportation, and information and referral (I&R) services.

Grants and donations play an important role in the funding of most adult day care programs. Fund raising is an ongoing effort for most program administrators. In addition, many programs charge fees, with participant fees covering more than 34 percent of the average budget. Fees typically range from $20 to $40, although a sliding scale based on income is often available. Families of older adults are sometimes willing to pay for day care because such services may allow a caretaker to work at a paying job that more than covers all fees. Private insurance does not cover most adult day care, although certain services may be reimbursable; insurers sometimes can be persuaded to pay for services on a case-by-case basis, particularly if it can be shown that adult day care is supplanting more expensive services. But private insurance coverage of adult day care is increasing.

Market: Most adult day care participants are over age 70 with some degree of physical or mental impairment. While they are unable to function completely independently, they do not require round-the-clock nursing care and are not bedridden. Some live alone, but a majority live with family members. Many adult day care clients suffer from chronic health problems that leave them unable to perform activities of daily living. Others are recovering from acute conditions, such as stroke or an injury, and need prolonged rehabilitative therapy. Still other individuals require therapeutic socialization and mental stimulation to retard or reverse the physical and mental decline that many older persons experience as a result of loneliness and isolation.

Estimating the market for adult day care is an inexact science. Two methods are commonly used. The demand method assumes that adult day care is a substitute for intermediate care, and, therefore, that methodologies appropriate for estimating intermediate care needs are rough indicators of demand for adult day care services. California, for example, assumes that about 5 percent of individuals over 65 need intermediate or adult day care services. The American Hospital Association estimates that 10 percent of acute care hospital discharges, 5 percent of nursing home discharges, and 1 percent of community residents are potential adult day care clients. However, some experts believe that only 25 percent of individuals needing the service are willing to use it. And of those who do use it, experience shows that few transfer directly from the hospital to day care. More typically they may be placed in day care after a period of stabilizing at home. Philip Weiler of the University of California at Davis estimates that current required service capacity for adult day care is less than seven places per thousand persons over age 65, and that potential required service capacity is no higher than fifteen places per thousand.

Another method for predicting demand for adult day care involves examining the local elderly population's health and social conditions. This requires gathering data on the number of persons over age 70, their living situations and income levels, and their capacity to perform activities of daily living. Nursing home occupancy rates, length of stay, and waitlist by reimbursement source must also be studied. In addition, this method requires data about the proportion of elderly acute care patients receiving health care referrals, as well as discharge information for home health care and homemaker programs.

Marketing: Marketing directly to potential adult day care clients is unlikely to be effective. A significant portion of day care participants suffer from senile dementia. Those who do not are often difficult to access or not trusting of persons they do not know.

Hospital discharge planners tend to be the best referral sources for adult day care programs and, therefore, should be contacted on a regular basis. Another excellent target is caregiver support groups, particularly those oriented toward Alzheimer's disease. Family members are the most likely decision-makers for adult day care placement. Community mental health providers should also be marketed, since few of them will have their own day care programs and, therefore, are more likely to be referral sources than competitors. Finally, physicians should be made aware of the program's presence and services.

Few adult day care programs have the budget to invest in promotional advertising. However, the service lends itself to public interest announcements or features in print and broadcast media. Press releases should be prepared and sent to local newspapers on a regular basis. The local area agency on aging should be aware of the existence and scope of day care services. Personnel divisions of large local businesses also should be contacted, since potential clients exist among both their retirees and, more frequently, the parents or older relatives of their current employees.

Most adult day care administrators find that one of their primary tasks involves public speaking to a variety of senior citizens' groups, either to raise funds or to publicize the program. In fact, these two goals are served by many of the same activities. Therefore, an important—though often underemphasized—skill for an adult day care manager is the ability to present the program well in group situations.

Competition: Direct competition for adult day care services comes primarily from community-based programs, as well as those sponsored by other local hospitals. The former are far more prevalent. Hospitals have significant competitive advantages and disadvantages vis-à-vis community-based programs. The larger institutions are better funded, have more reliable reputations, enjoy better access to medical care, and have natural referral sources via their own discharge planners. However, hospitals also tend to have substantially higher costs, particularly in terms of staff, who are paid roughly 50 percent more for the same jobs in a hospital-sponsored program versus a community-based service.

In the future, a growing source of competition (or of subcontracted participants) may be corporate-sponsored programs. Corporations are beginning to look at adult day care as an employee benefit, but so far only a few corporations have entered the field with pilot programs.

Timetable: The time needed to establish an adult day care center depends partly on regulation and location. Licensure and certification procedures may take several months to complete. A program requiring construction or renovation will take longer to initiate than one simply moving into an existing structure. Arranging transportation, purchasing furniture, and refitting the physical space with safety rails and other fixtures for the disabled can be accomplished in a matter of weeks, if necessary. Most adult day care centers can be ready to open within a few months, but premarketing should start well ahead of time if the program is to start with a good-sized census. It is difficult to get a stable client population. Though there are waiting lists in some areas, in other areas it may take up to two years to reach the enrollment goal, which can strain the financial viability of the operation.

Management: Adult day care can be managed in several ways. A hospital can establish and operate its own program. It can team with a community provider to offer day care services, bringing greater combined resources to the program but raising potential disagreements due to differences in philosophy. Third, a hospital can merely support a community-based program without becoming heavily involved in day-to-day operations.

A hospital considering sponsoring an adult day care program must identify its motives before determining its management strategy. The institution aiming to establish and control an integrated eldercare service spectrum might choose to develop its own program, whereas one that is more concerned about ensuring the availability of the service might prefer to form a supportive relationship with an existing community-based provider. If the objective is to enhance visibility and bring adult day care into the hospital referral network, any situation that affiliates the institution with a day care program may meet the need.

Development Concerns: At least 25 to 40 square feet of space per patient is recommended as a minimum facility requirement. Ideally, a program should have at least 1250 to 1500 square feet to serve 25 persons. Specialized Alzheimer's units will require somewhat more room. The bulk of the space, perhaps 75 percent, will be used for patient care. The rest will be used for staff offices, storage, bathrooms, and perhaps kitchen facilities. Ideally, the patient care area should be a single large room divisible by movable partitions into several small rooms for maximum flexibility.

Most regulations governing adult day care programs derive from state authority and vary by state. States may require licensure or certification, both, or neither. Medicare has no certification process, and states may or may not require certification for programs receiving Medicaid reimbursement. Most states have some form of standards governing staffing, organization, facilities, and services for adult day care programs. The local AAA or SUA can provide information about state regulations.

Most adult day care programs serve between 10 and 100 persons, although average daily census generally ranges between 30 and 50 percent of participants. Nationwide, the average daily census is 24 persons; optimal average daily census is about 40 persons.

Information Sources: The National Institute for Adult Daycare (NIAD), a branch of the National Council on Aging, is located at 600 Maryland Avenue, S.W., Suite 208W—West Wing, Washington, DC 20024; (202) 479-1200. The NIAD has a wealth of information and publications about funding, staffing, developing, and marketing adult day care programs, as well as up-to-date information about national standards and regulations. Their book, *Adult Daycare in America: Summary of a National Survey* (1986), may be ordered for $6.00. An in-depth analysis of the data from the national survey is scheduled for publication at the end of 1988. *The Directory of Adult Daycare in America,* a 1987 state-by-state listing of all day care programs, is available for $19.95 (plus $2.00 shipping and handling). State day care organizations and SUAs can supply pertinent state and local regulations and funding information.

The American Hospital Association's affiliated Office on Aging and Long-Term Care published a 16-page topic report on adult day care in 1983. Now slightly dated, it is nonetheless a useful guide. The booklet sells for under $10 and can be ordered from The Hospital Research and Educational Trust, 840 North Lake Shore Drive, Chicago, IL 60611; (312) 280-6382.

Aging Resource Centers

Two of the greatest health needs of older people are access to information and access to services provided in the community. Older adults have powerful incentives to get the best information they can, because the consequences of not becoming informed on health issues are potentially great: illness, dependency, institutionalization, and early death. The older population faces a maze of providers, payers, and celebrities, all hawking various products. The information offered is often contradictory and of dubious credibility.

Similarly, older adults' access to the services offered in their own communities is often limited by simple ignorance of what is available. Older people want to make good choices about their health, yet they are seldom presented with clear, complete, and dependable information on which to base those choices. Practical information and resources that are accessible, easy to understand, and of the highest credibility are critical to the mental and physical well-being of older persons.

Nor is it only older people who are interested in information about health and aging and access to the community's resources. Adult children and other caregivers have indicated in surveys a desire for instruction and direction in caring for aging relatives or friends.

Physicians and other providers, many of whom find themselves treating more older than younger persons, require clinical information on the special needs of an aging body and mind. Organizations and individuals involved in the aging network need to know about national and local policies and issues.

An aging resource center is designed to meet the information needs of a community's older adults, their caregivers, providers, advocates, and others with an interest in the elderly. Resource centers provide comprehensive collections of information on issues and organizations pertaining to health, wellness, care needs, and lifestyle. An aging resource center may also include information about legal and financial issues as well as leisure pursuits. A center may contain books, magazines, pamphlets, films, and video materials on subjects relating to the well-being and vitality of older adults, as well as books, journals, and related publications pertaining to geriatric medicine and the clinical care of the elderly.

Far more than a library, a club, a continuing education program, or a storefront help center, the aging resource center combines all these to become a social center, the hub of the local eldercare network and the living human interface between the hospital and one of its major constituencies. An aging resource center combines:

- the best information, aimed at the public, on health, wellness and aging, whether books, pamphlets, videos, or magazines;

- the best information for the clinician;

- health screenings and health fairs;

- referral and counseling for health, wellness and life-style issues;

- exercise and wellness programs;

- support groups;

- community meeting space;

- educational programs and speakers; and

- social events.

The most successful resource centers are driven by their programs, not by their collections of information. Franciscan Health System in Cincinnati, for instance, links its resource center, called Senior Network, with the OASIS senior outreach program sponsored by the May Department Stores Company and its foundation. Their educational program mixes courses on nutrition, Alzheimer's disease, and diabetes with travel evenings, lessons on the dulcimer, and instruction in T'ai Chi. Some resource centers offer social evenings, bingo, group tours, and interest exchanges where a bridge threesome might find a fourth or a guitar picker might find a fiddle player.

These dynamic program mixes generate the interest and traffic that feed into the hospital's eldercare program. The center often turns out to be the most fertile recruiting ground for the hospital's senior membership program.

An aging resource center can be located either on or off the hospital campus. Because the objective is community involvement in a hospital-based program, an argument can be made for either location. However, most hospitals choose to locate the aging resource center offsite, since many prospective users indicate a reluctance to enter hospitals except when absolutely necessary. Some institutions separate the staff library (for use by clinicians and administrators) and keep that onsite with the existing hospital library, and put the community-oriented components of the resource center offsite. The community center typically requires up to 2000 square feet of space, including offices, library areas, and meeting rooms. The Franciscan Health System Senior Network, for instance, is located in a retirement complex. Mother Frances Hospital's LifeWorks in Tyler, Texas, takes up 1000 square feet in the Broadway Mall.

Value: An aging resource center provides a variety of benefits to older persons, their caregivers, providers, and the sponsoring hospital. Older people gain from having a central source of information about health, wellness, life-style, and other pertinent issues. The center assists sick persons in recovery, well individuals in maintaining and improving health, and everyone in learning about issues of general interest to older persons. Some centers provide health insurance counseling to guide older people through the maze of payment plans and bills.

The resource center can provide a wide variety of information and network links almost instantly. The Vintage Health Library and Resource Center at Alta Bates-Herrick Hospital in Berkeley, California, for instance, fielded a frantic call from a woman whose 82-year-old mother in Santa Monica was being harassed and threatened by drug dealers who had taken over her building. Calling the police had only increased the level of threat. The Vintage Center connected her with the right elder housing concerns in Los Angeles, and her mother had a new home that night.

An aging resource center is a place for older people to learn about and discuss issues that affect them with others of similar interests. The resource center serves as a social and informational hub for the older community.

Caregivers use the aging resource center to become informed about the illnesses from which their relatives, friends, or patients suffer. In addition, the center provides information about the delivery of care and the special needs of those looking after older people. Some elder service managers believe that the heaviest users of the resource centers are adult children of older people.

Providers benefit from having on hand the most up-to-date information about geriatric services. Since relatively few physicians are specifically trained in geriatrics, a collection of the best medical books and current journals detailing clinical and research information about older people is particularly helpful. In addition, physicians can refer elderly patients to the aging resource center in order to clarify or underscore issues involved with causes and treatment of health conditions, or to provide access to the network of eldercare services available locally.

Hospitals benefit from developing an aging resource center as much as their constituents and providers. If, because of its demographics and its vision of the future, a hospital wants eldercare to become one of its "centers of excellence," it can hardly do without some kind of aging resource center that will:

- connect it directly to large numbers of older people and those who care about and for them;

- put it in direct daily interchange with all the service providers in the aging network;

- give it, as well as its constituents, the best information available about healthy aging; and

- project in the community the idea that the hospital is the leading institution for eldercare in the area.

A resource center is an excellent marketing tool, providing a means to attract not only the older persons who have been to the hospital, but also the caregivers of older people and the well elderly seeking to maintain their health. Up to several thousand visits will be made to the center over the course of a year, and media coverage of the opening and ongoing special events is relatively easy to attract.

A resource center can attract not only more patients, but a better mix of patients. An aging resource center can place a hospital squarely in the center of the aging network in its community, providing a basis of collaboration with local agencies and individuals. Finally, a center is an ideal project for soliciting financial support from community organization and individual donors.

Cost: The capital costs of an aging resource center depend on its location and comprehensiveness. A center located inside a hospital will require material and development costs ranging from $150,000 to $200,000. Construction or renovation of an offsite facility can add significantly to expenditures, depending upon the square footage and the services and programs offered. Furniture, supplies, and additional equipment may increase costs by $20,000 to $50,000. Staff library material and development expenditures typically range from $10,000 to $30,000.

Operating costs depend largely on staffing. Resource centers using volunteers for most tasks will keep operating costs to a minimum. Although a professional librarian usually oversees the information at the center, some hospitals use their staff librarians to manage the information at both facilities. Onsite resource centers carry a portion of hospital overhead, but require few additional expenditures other than staffing.

Staffing: The programs that the aging resource center supports will, of course, dictate its staffing needs. Mother Frances Hospital's mall center in Tyler, Texas, for instance, offers walk-in health screenings, so its center is staffed by an RN whenever the mall is open.

For an aging resource center to be successful, its manager may be an RN or a social worker, but she or he must be someone who is experienced in the eldercare network.

An emphasis on dynamic programming requires a strong volunteer commitment. But that very programming can generate the kind of interest, community involvement, and traffic that makes it easier to draw volunteers from beyond the hospital's traditional volunteer pool.

Some hospitals use their staff librarians to oversee both the information at the resource center and the inhouse staff facility. Paid staff can be supplemented with retired librarians from the community and other volunteers, perhaps students from local colleges. Many older persons who are reluctant to volunteer in a hospital environment are eager to donate their time to a resource center.

Beyond merely coordinating books and other materials, staff are needed to assist visitors in finding and using information. Resource centers with bookstore components that also serve as information and referral centers require knowledgeable personnel—usually volunteers—to answer phones and to provide referrals and health insurance counseling. These positions can provide interesting opportunities to skilled volunteers seeking new challenges within the hospital.

Revenues: The primary way the aging resource center generates revenue is by strategically positioning it as the center of the local aging network and the leader in eldercare in its region.

There are ways that a resource center can generate revenues directly, but they are minor, and it is not to be expected that such revenues will cover the center's operating costs. For instance, while no reimbursement is available for a center's core services, some associated services, such as case management or certain types of health education, may be eligible for some public or private third-party funding. Though none of the current centers charge fees, it might be possible to charge for individual memberships, loan privileges, research packages, community resource counseling, health insurance counseling, or tape rentals. If a bookstore component were added, sales of books, tapes, and posters might generate from several hundred to several thousand dollars in annual revenues. A number of the existing centers do charge for such professional services as health screenings, as well as for courses.

A much more interesting idea is that an aging resource center is an excellent vehicle for soliciting financial support from foundations, organizations, local businesses, and individual donors. The center's visibility in the community, the wide publicity it attracts, and its progressive, wellness-oriented image combine to make the facility an ideal project on which to base fund-raising. Local businesses that attract older customers also may be interested in subsidizing furniture or equipment. The relative newness of the resource center concept also adds to its publicity generating and fund-raising potential. Some or all of the capital costs for the project may be covered by donations.

The center's fund-raising work can be directly tied in to the hospital's own, putting it in direct contact with healthy older people, potential donors, who might not otherwise be easily reached, and providing a positive, visible project with which local corporations would be pleased to identify.

In Louisville, for instance, Jewish Hospital carefully developed a relationship with locally based Kentucky Fried Chicken. The hospital had been Colonel Sanders' hospital until his death. When opening a new geriatric wing, the hospital asked the corporation's permission to name it after Colonel Sanders, as an active, dynamic older American, without asking for a donation. They asked the Colonel's widow to cut the ribbon for the new wing, put a bust of the Colonel across from the nurse's station, involved the corporation in activities at the hospital, and kept the corporation informed. When the hospital decided to develop an aging resource center, it asked for and got a $125,000 contribution for what became the Colonel Sanders Geriatric Center.

Market: A major pitfall in the development of an aging resource center is to conceive its market too narrowly, as consisting only of fairly frail senior citizens. The center's wealth of programs and illness- and wellness-oriented information is of potential interest to all mature adults, that is, those over age 45 or 50. In fact, Mother Frances Hospital decided not to put anything in the name or marketing material of LifeWorks that would say it was for any particular age group.

The market for an aging resource center has four segments: (1) older people, (2) their caretakers, (3) providers, and (4) community organizations. Some elder service directors report that the largest market for their resource center is the adult children of older parents, who seek information about their parents' ailments and community resources to assist with the duties of caretaking.

Providers may choose to use either the staff or community component of the aging resource center and may recommend that their older patients and caretakers use the community center. Making physicians and pharmacists aware of the center and of the specific materials it contains facilitates the referral process. Community organizations also represent potential referral sources, as well as potential users. Additionally, community groups may provide staff assistance or may offer to house their organizational resource collections in the center.

Marketing: The center is marketed through its programs. Those programs are usually best marketed through existing networks, such as churches, doctors' offices, the hospital itself, the local area agency on aging, the local chapter of the American Association of Retired Persons (AARP), senior centers, nutrition programs, and local community colleges and continuing education programs, which often boast very high enrollment of older people.

Public service announcements in the media can have excellent results. When they are offering a specific benefit, such as a health screening, some resource centers have gotten very good mileage out of paid ads in local media.

The premarketing of an aging resource center can dovetail with the selection of the information materials to be included. Older persons, providers, and interested community groups can be solicited for input about broad themes and specific books and journals. Representatives can be invited to review audiovisual materials prior to their purchase. Questionnaires asking for input, sent to interested parties, serve to elicit feedback, enhance visibility, and arouse interest in the center.

The aging resource center can be promoted in a number of ways. An opening event can attract wide television, radio, and print media coverage. Appropriate individuals should be invited to this and to regularly scheduled open houses. Government and community publications pertaining to older people can include information about the center. Older people themselves can be contacted as inpatients through discharge planners.

Providers, especially physicians, should be courted as referral sources. The fragmentation of the aging network leaves most older people confused about where to go for help; typically, they turn to their physician for answers. By inviting physicians to special events and keeping them and their office staffs informed through mailings or a newsletter, an aging resource center can develop what may become its best referral channels. Physicians can be made aware of standard information packages on common conditions, such as arthritis and heart disease, and can then literally write an "information prescription" for their patients to take to the aging resource center to have "filled."

An aging resource center must be designed for easy public access and comfortable reading and gathering. Ideally, the center should be located on a building's ground floor, with convenient parking, ramps, and doors that are easy to open or that open automatically. Proximity to public transportation is critical. Doors, signs, hallways, and toilet facilities all should be designed with an eye to the special needs of older people.

Competition: You are not likely to have any competition. And if you develop a center, you are likely to preempt any competition. Most hospitals have floundered in their attempts to form a coherent eldercare strategy, because they have lacked this critical link between them, their constituents, and the aging network. At this writing, no communities have more than one center, and most have none. Even health resource centers directed at all ages are rare.

Indirect competition may come from information and referral centers and from case management agencies. However, it is more likely that such entities would serve as referral sources than as competition. Public or university libraries and local bookstores may offer some competition in terms of books and journals, but a dedicated aging resource center is likely to be more comprehensive, specific, and dynamic, with programs that forge a direct link with the community. YMCAs, Jewish community centers, churches, and other organizations that have a traditional strong link with older people should be viewed not as competition but as partners and sources of referrals. General libraries also are likely to be excellent referral channels.

While most areas presently do not have aging resource centers, small and medium-size communities may not have the client traffic to support more than one. Thus, the hospital that initially establishes a center may effectively preclude its competitors from doing so. The time and expertise necessary to develop an aging resource center and the linkages formed with providers and community organizations may give the hospital first developing a center an advantage in the eldercare market that is difficult to overcome.

Timetable: The time required to establish an aging resource center depends largely on two issues: the development process and the nature of the facility. A hospital that uses its own librarian or a knowledgeable gerontological researcher may need 12 to 24 months to identify, locate, order, and catalog all books and other materials. This timetable will be shortened considerably if the resource center is purchased as a turnkey operation from a development consultant. In that case, materials can be selected and ordered in a matter of a few months, depending on the desired amount of input from the hospital and community.

In a turnkey situation, construction and renovation needs may determine how soon the resource center can be opened. If a suitable space is available, operations can begin soon after materials are received and furniture and equipment are purchased—perhaps five or six months altogether. Significant refurbishment or construction can add four to twelve months to the process.

Management: An aging resource center typically is managed by a coordinator, overseen by a hospital's director of elder services. The management is rarely contracted out or joint-ventured. The required expertise usually is present within the existing hospital staff, although thorough knowledge of geriatrics and gerontology generally is not available. Because the number of trained gerontological librarians in the country is very small, an experienced consultant often is hired to help select the materials and develop the center, but the hospital itself will manage the project.

Development Concerns: Whether or not your institution should develop an aging resource center depends on how you see the future of health care. If eldercare is an important part of that future, if access to the older market is important, and if the public perception of your institution as the leader in eldercare within your region is important, then an aging resource center may have a key role in building toward that future. Many hospital planners anticipate that the health care system of the future will be some type of capitated, case management model, at the heart of which will be information and referral services. Establishing an aging resource center may position sponsoring institutions to take the lead in the emerging eldercare system.

Hospitals also believe that they reap significant marketing benefits from developing an aging resource center. The newness of the concept helps position these hospitals as national leaders or innovators in eldercare and community service. Significantly, the institutions sponsoring aging resource centers typically are among the nation's most respected hospitals and medical centers.

Information Sources: For further information about a working resource center, contact LifeWorks at Mother Frances Hospital in Tyler, Texas. The resource center itself is at 4651 South Broadway, Broadway Mall, Tyler, TX 75703; (214) 561-6255. Another aging resource center is the Center for 55+ , Hillcrest Hospital, 3220 South Peoria Avenue, Tulsa, OK 74105; (918) 744-5595.

The major aging resource center development consultant is Age Wave®, Inc., at 1900 Powell Street, Suite 800, Emeryville, CA 94608; (415) 652-9099.

Case Management

Case management is an array of services that helps individuals find and receive appropriate care. The spectrum of potential services for the elderly is large, fragmented, and often confusing. Most older adults and their families are unaware of the breadth of that spectrum, the services that are available locally, where those services can be found, and what sources will pay for them. Therefore, a centralized coordination function is at the core of an effective eldercare program.

The term "case management" can be confusing. As eldercare has mushroomed in recent years, it has come to be used for a variety of functions that are quite distinct, and which sometimes even operate at cross purposes. Within the hospital setting there are four versions of the term:

1. *Traditional management* of medical cases is aimed at obtaining the best treatment for the patient.

2. *Cost-control-driven management* of medical cases, also called "utilization management," has the goal of delivering the appropriate but least expensive care to the patient.

3. *Hospital discharge planning* since the institution of DRGs, has changed from seeing that the patient is comfortable and provided for on returning home to managing extensive use of high-tech equipment, caregiving and regimens for keeping the patient's condition stable, such as IV therapy, physical therapy, and special nutritional therapy.

4. *Geriatric case management,* while hospital-based, may not be the result of any acute episode in which the client was hospitalized. This type of management coordinates services available in the community, and may cover anything that an elderly person might need to stay out of an institution, from nursing care to getting the lawns mowed and the shutters painted.

These four types of case management all specifically include medical assessment, and are an extension of the hospital's traditional function.

A fifth variation, *private geriatric case management*, often includes managing therapies, but specifically leaves out any medical assessment or prescription. Rather than an extension of the hospital's traditional function, it is a privatization of the social worker's function. But hospitals can enter this rapidly growing field, and many have. Unlike medical case management, which is necessary but usually only profitable to the extent that it controls costs, this social case management can often be profitable. In fact, over 65 percent of the private firms that engage in it are for-profit.

Terminology can be further confused by marketing considerations: case management, while fairly descriptive from the provider standpoint, is resented by some patients who do not want their cases "managed." Therefore, many programs are using other nomenclatures, the most common of which is *care coordination.*

We will be discussing primarily the last two types of case management, which project beyond the hospital into the community, using community resources in an attempt to help the client stay independent. But all five types of case management do have a number of elements in commmon:

- *case finding*, to reach individuals needing help;

- *prescreening and assessment*, to determine who most requires help and what those needs are;

- *care planning*, to coordinate an individualized array of services and supportive activities;

- *monitoring utilization*, to develop a database on the population being served and to report to government agencies and private payers; and

- *reassessment*, to evaluate the suitability and effectiveness of the care plan on an ongoing basis and to modify or terminate it as needed.

Another element of case management involves assessing client and family financial resources and determining and helping to arrange a means to pay for care coordination services.

Hospital-based case management programs vary widely in size

and scope. Some have staffs as large as 20, including administrators, case managers, and support personnel. On the other end of the spectrum, though, Middlesex Memorial Hospital in Middletown, Connecticut, has a well-regarded case management program that employs just one social worker for all administrative and clinical functions. Size is not a requirement of a successful program: nearly all of the hundreds of private case management firms around the country consist of just one or two persons. Service breadth may involve only assessment and care arrangement, or may include case finding, information and referral, individual and family counseling, ongoing care monitoring, financial guidance, and a host of other services.

There are two basic models of case management for long-term care. One of these is known as the *brokerage model*, in which the case management entity arranges care from available service providers, but does not itself supply any services. Huntington Memorial Hospital's Senior Care Network (see Case Study 5 in Chapter 4) is a brokered program. The other major model, the much less common *consolidated direct services model*, involves a central agency that provides all or nearly all needed services through its own resources. Perhaps the best known example of this model is the On Lok Community Care Organization for Dependent Adults in San Francisco.

Typically, case management works this way: an older adult is recommended as a potential client by the family or by a health professional and is brought to the hospital for an assessment. A clinical team screens and examines the patient to gauge health needs and to determine whether care coordination services are required. If so, a case manager begins to work with the client and family to develop a care plan, which consists of needed services and support activities. This professional contacts local providers, who may or may not be formally affiliated with the hospital. The case manager arranges for services and advises the family on how best to proceed. He or she also keeps in touch with the client and family on an ongoing basis to monitor service utilization and health status, and periodically reassesses client needs, rearranging the care plan as necessary.

Most private case management firms offer a complete range of services, including:

- functional, social, and financial assessment;

- planning, referring, and coordinating services;

- monitoring the delivery of services;

- evaluating whether or not the client needs to be placed in an institution; and

- assisting the client to complete forms.

The services they provide most frequently are counseling for the family or caregiver, counseling for the client, and placement in a nursing home or other appropriate housing.

Value: Case management helps guide the frail elderly through the disjointed long-term care system to the appropriate level of care. Few older persons are familiar with the services that are available in their community or the appropriateness of those services to their needs. Case managers help older adults by identifying their needs, determining a care plan, coordinating services, and suggesting or arranging financing mechanisms.

Case management can be tremendously beneficial to families living far from older relatives. Over one-fourth of adults live at least 100 miles from their parents, making either direct care or service arrangement difficult. A case management program can take responsibility for assessing needs and coordinating all care, saving either the adult child or the older parent from relocating.

Hospitals benefit from offering case management in a number of respects. The service meets an important community need and has a positive impact on institutional reputation. It can be a powerful public relations tool, especially because few hospitals currently offer the service. Case management may represent an additional referral source if clients are referred to hospital-affiliated services, such as skilled nursing facilities, home health care, or adult day care.

Hospitals that offer care coordination services may gain an advantage over their competitors in the long run, as the eldercare system evolves. As the spectrum of reimbursable services broadens to include nonacute care, it will become increasingly important for hospitals to know where and how that care can be provided. Those institutions already familiar with the aging network will be better prepared to provide or contract for long-term care. In addition, as health care reimbursement moves toward capitation, hospitals experienced in care coordination will be best able to provide quality care efficiently by ensuring that patients are in the least intensive service level that is appropriate.

Cost: Case management usually is not a profitable service, and most programs are heavily subsidized. Assessment, which typically involves an hour or two of a physician's time, is especially costly. However, an organization that provides ongoing care, as in a consolidated direct services model, may be able to recoup a good portion of the funds expended on assessment services.

Labor accounts for the dominant costs involved in a case management program, and thus operating expenses are largely dependent on staff size. A typical program with 2.5 FTEs will cost approximately $100,000 in salaries and overhead expenses. A hospital-based case management service with 3.5 FTEs will have operating expenses of approximately $125,000. Case managers generally earn between $20,000 and $35,000 annually.

Capital costs need not be substantial. Programs can be housed in existing hospital office space. The only new capital expense might be computer hardware and software to keep abreast of community resources, track cases, and store information. A personal computer costing as little as $1000 can suffice. Case management software is in its infancy. United Seniors Health Cooperative of Washington, D.C., has developed a case management software package called Benefits Eligibility. With this program, basic information about the person is input into the computer, with the resulting output listing community and government services for which the person is eligible.

Case finding is inexpensive for a hospital-sponsored case management program, since the majority of long-term care cases begin with hospitalization. Patients with intensive or unusual needs require care coordination that is perhaps twice as expensive as those patients with more typical needs.

Staffing: As noted above, hospital-sponsored case management programs may have staffs as large as twenty or as small as one. Since most programs currently offered are relatively new, they tend to be small, typically about 2.5 FTEs. This would include a case manager, an administrator, and a half-time secretary. The administrator spends up to half of his or her time managing cases and the rest supervising the program.

Although staff come from a variety of backgrounds, administrators tend to be social workers, and case managers often hold nursing or social work degrees. Some programs operate under the philosophy that case management is best performed by nurses, especially the assessment function. Others believe that although discharge planning is a nursing function, care coordination is essentially a social service and, therefore, is best handled by social workers. Still others allow trained volunteers to manage most elements of care coordination.

Each case manager can handle up to 40 clients per week, although 30 is perhaps the optimal figure. This generally translates into an average caseload of between 300 and 400 clients. However, the caseload mix will affect the demands made on case managers. Very ill clients or those needing hard-to-find services take far more time than mildly disabled clients needing readily available care. In a typical case mix, client needs will average three to four hours per month. Severely ill clients will require seven to eight hours per month until their conditions stabilize.

Revenues: Revenues for case management services come either from government programs or private fees charged to clients. Overall, much care coordination is performed at low or no charge by area agencies on aging, community organizations, religious groups, senior centers, or hospitals.

At this point in time, reimbursement for case management services is so limited that virtually all programs are subsidized. However, hospital-sponsored fee-for-service programs aimed at upper-middle class individuals and families are appearing around the country, and many hope to break even in the near future. Typical charges range from $50 to $75 per hour, but vary according to several factors:

- where the consultation takes place (inhome visits are more costly than office conferences);
- case complexity;

- the number of consultations (clients receiving more services may be charged less per consultation); and

- whether the visit is an initial or subsequent consultation (initial meetings are more expensive).

At $60 to $70 per hour, an ambitious program might raise $100,000 in annual revenues, but this has yet to be demonstrated. In addition, many programs charge fees on a sliding scale based on income. However, such fees rarely defray operating costs to any significant degree.

The most common private rate is $50 per hour, with or without a sliding fee. Most of these payments are made out of pocket by the client or the client's caregivers.

At present, although hospitals have been able to attract clients willing to pay substantial fees, full fee-for-service volume is not great enough to cover program costs. Many essential service elements, including some research and all marketing, are not billable to clients. Table 3-1 demonstrates the billable hours necessary for a fee-for-service case management program to break even financially. Assuming 3.5 FTEs generating $125,000 in annual operating expenses and providing 2.25 FTEs of care coordination services at $60 per hour, billable hours would need to average almost 19 hours a week per case manager FTE to achieve breakeven. This implies a successful marketing effort.

TABLE 3-1
Breakeven Calculation for Case Management Program

Operating costs for 3.5 FTEs	$125,000
Weekly revenue needed (125,000 ÷ 50)	$ 2500
Weekly revenue per FTE (2500 ÷ 2.25*)	$ 1111.11
Weekly billable hours needed per FTE per week at $60 per hour ($1111.11 ÷ 60)	18.51

*Actual case management = 2.25 FTEs.

Private social case management typically focuses specifically on services that are not usually reimbursable through Medicare, Medicaid, or other public programs. For-profit programs will refer those unable to pay to less comprehensive, but lower cost, community programs.

Some hospital-based programs are structured to gain maximum reimbursement from Medicare. At University Hospitals of Cleveland's Geriatric CARE Center, nursing and social work fees are billed as technical charges with overhead so that Medicare will reimburse expenses. Medicare and supplemental insurance cover most diagnostic assessment services performed by a physician, who often agrees to accept assignment. Although reimbursement does not come close to covering expenses, this structure does defray a portion of the cost of care planning and case monitoring.

Market: The market for case management services are the frail, dependent elderly and their families. Most programs have minimum age requirements ranging from 55 to 65. Younger persons with severe chronic disabilities may also benefit from these services. Certain categories of elders are particularly strong candidates for case management, including those recovering from strokes and major-joint procedures, and those suffering from cancer, degenerative neurological conditions, or other complex problems. Because case management is an expensive service to provide for most patients, the target population should be carefully defined in advance so that only those who could truly benefit will be served.

Although case management itself is expensive, case finding is relatively inexpensive for a hospital-based program. Because a large proportion of patients with serious chronic problems are hospitalized at some point, a hospital can identify potential clients before discharge and, often, at point of entry. In addition, some calls to a hospital's information and referral service can be referred to a case manager.

Hospitals usually do not conduct surveys of market demand for case management services. Nearly all communities suffer from a lack of such services, or at least a lack of adequately funded services. Where case management has been made available, both older adults and their families have expressed strong interest in enrolling. Nevertheless, hospitals intending to establish fee-for-service case management programs would be wise to determine if enough potential volume exists to support such programs. This is an area for which little reliable market forecast data is available.

Marketing: There are four major markets at whom case management programs should be targeted: (1) potential patients and their families, (2) local providers, (3) financial and legal trustees, and (4) community organizations. Patients can be contacted while hospitalized or during elder health fairs. Adult children of the elderly can be notified of case management services through caregiver support networks or through the human resource departments of their employers. Hospitals might advertise in the yellow pages of major metropolitan centers outside of their service areas to promote case management services to adult children who live far from their parents.

Hospital discharge planners, including those affiliated with other hospitals that lack case management programs, can be excellent referral sources. They should be informed of the program and new developments. Physicians, especially those with a large number of chronically ill patients, also represent referral sources. In addition, social workers and mental health professionals should be notified of case management services. Lawyers and bank trust officers often are called upon to act as guardians of or advisors to older adults and their families, and, thus, may be in positions to recommend case management services. For all of these groups, open houses may be useful as promotional vehicles, but direct mail is likely to reach a larger number of busy professionals.

Community organizations, including senior groups, service agencies, and religious institutions, also should be contacted. Most case management program supervisors make regular public presentations to local groups and agencies to publicize their services. These organizations can be kept informed by direct mailings, some of which might include posters or other visual reminders of the program.

Private case managers rarely receive referrals from those in public programs. Usually the referrals go the other direction: private managers refer clients who cannot afford their services. The private managers typically rely on physicians and other clients for referrals. The clients that these private case managers serve are not that different from the rest of the typical population in their age group. The typical private client is a widow in her late seventies or early eighties, living alone, with an annual income of $5000 to $15,000.

One potential appeal to the children of aging parents is the possibility of claiming case management fees as tax deductions. Older adults may be claimed as dependents by their children if their income is under $1080 (excluding Social Security payments) and if the child pays for more than half the cost of support (including Social Security) for the entire year, even if the older person is living alone. There is a possibility that case management fees for an elderly dependent may be tax-deductible as medical expenses; however, to date no relevant case has yet been adjudicated by any tax court.

Competition: Private, fee-for-service case management is a rapidly growing field of many tiny firms, most of whom have been in business for three years or less. A majority are independent. Others are affiliated with hospitals, social service agencies or nursing homes.

On the other hand, as with most unprofitable long-term care services, there is relatively little competition among subsidized hospital-sponsored case management programs. A recent survey of community hospitals by the American Hospital Association found that less than 3 percent of respondents offered case management services for the elderly. The most significant competition that hospital-sponsored programs are likely to feel comes from community agencies.

Area agencies on aging, senior centers, charitable groups, religious organizations, and community agencies may offer case management services. A survey in San Francisco found nearly 15 programs, only one of which was associated with a hospital. These services often are provided at no charge, although in some cases a sliding scale is offered. Eligibility requirements vary widely: the most common restrictions involve area of residence, Medicaid eligibility, affiliation with the sponsoring organization, gender, or psychological needs. Clients often have limited financial resources.

Hospitals should be careful about competing with community organizations. These groups often have been coordinating care for years, probably do it well, and often have some sort of constituency. Hospitals may rely on some of these seemingly competitive organizations to provide needed long-term or personal care services.

An effort should be made to avoid duplication of case management services, especially since most communities lack sufficient capabilities in this regard. The hospital that succeeds in bringing together various community agencies and develops a system that most efficiently uses local resources is providing a unique and very valuable service to its community.

Some physicians perceive themselves to be in the case management business. They assess health needs, counsel patients and families, and recommend appropriate care. Professional case managers tend to be better informed than physicians about available care options and are in better positions to monitor service and revise care planning. Nevertheless, it is important for hospital-based case management programs to realize the danger of being perceived as competing with physicians.

Other competition may come from a growing number of small proprietary firms. A typical firm has two case managers, usually social workers or mental health professionals. They work on a fee-for-service basis only, and usually bill their services at $60 to $75 per hour. Sometimes a flat fee of about $250 is charged for comprehensive assessment, care plan, and service arrangement or referral. Little reliable information is available on the hundreds of such firms scattered around the country. However, InterStudy (a Minnesota-based, not-for-profit research and consulting organization), has just released a study funded by the Retirement Research Foundation that examines all aspects of private geriatric case management.

In general, hospitals enjoy distinct advantages over their competitors when operating case management programs. As noted above, case finding is far easier and less expensive for hospitals than for other organizations. In addition, hospitals generally have more credibility than other agencies in the eyes of the community when it comes to providing health care services. Finally, the hospital discharge planner and medical staff offer important referral sources that are less inclined to recommend competing community-based case management programs.

Timetable: The time involved in establishing a case management program depends largely on program size and scope. Nonetheless, all programs share certain characteristics. Some degree of premarketing is important so that a program has clients when the doors open. However, because a large proportion of clients come from the inpatient population, premarketing is less critical for case management than for many other services.

Case managers in a brokerage model program will require time to gain familiarity with local providers. The time involved will depend on the size and complexity of the aging network and the background of the staff. Because many case managers have backgrounds in discharge planning, social work, or community service agencies, time required for this task often is minimal.

Patient and utilization tracking are important to a case management program, and information systems usually are established to facilitate these tasks. However, the systems have not always been in service at the start of a program. Paper records can be sufficient for a small service until hardware and software are in place.

Many of the early case management programs often took a year or more to plan. More recent services take far less time, since viable models are now available to emulate. A typical smaller case management program can be operational within a few months of its inception.

Development Concerns: Regulation is not a major concern in case management. Other than the licensing requirements of the various professionals employed, there are very few state or federal regulations that apply to case management, particularly private, nonmedical case management.

But an important factor in the success of a medical case management program is physician acceptance. Physicians may be uninterested in, or even threatened by, this service if they understand it as management of a patient's health needs. Emphasis should be placed on the distinction between management of clinical medical needs and coordination of broader health and social support services. Physicians should feel comfortable with the authority that case managers hold and should be kept informed of significant changes in a patient's health status and care plan. Physicians also should be encouraged to take advantage of case managers' knowledge about available community resources.

Hospitals seeking ways to make their case management programs profitable might attempt to contract with corporations for a variety of services. Businesses are quite concerned about skyrocketing health care costs for their retired employees and generally are interested in any serious efforts to manage those costs. A hospital, in conjunction with a third-party payer, might try designing a pre-retirement package that includes case management services as a cost control measure—although most such packages currently available involve more utilization control than true case management. Case management expertise and knowledge also could be marketed for counseling current employees who are caring for aging relatives.

Information Sources: The American Hospital Association publishes a monograph entitled *Case Management: Issues for Hospitals,* catalog number 501011, for $8.50. It includes information about establishing a hospital-based case management program, as well as some brief case studies and a recommended bibliography. The publication is available from the American Hospital Association, 840 North Lake Shore Drive, Chicago, IL 60611; (312) 280-6030.

On Lok Senior Health Services, a remarkably successful capitated program serving the frail elderly of San Francisco's Chinatown, provides a wide range of consulting services for organizations interested in developing their own such programs; part of their expertise involves case management. The consulting service can be reached at On Lok, 1441 Powell Street, San Francisco, CA 94133; (415) 989-2578.

Middlesex Memorial Hospital is another good source of information about case management. Contact Middlesex Memorial Hospital, Middletown, CT 06457; (203) 347-9471.

A good example of hospital-based private case management is Elderplan at Mount Zion Medical Center in San Francisco. It is part of a broad continuum of services provided for the elderly through the hospital's Institute on Aging. Elderplan attempts to help its clients stay independent whenever possible. Case managers visit the home to conduct functional and social assessments, then consult family members to ascertain financial resources before making recommendations for services. Contact the Institute on Aging, P.O. Box 7921, San Francisco, CA 94120; (415) 885-7800.

The most comprehensive source of information on private care management is the 1987 InterStudy report on 117 firms. Titled *Private Care Management,* by Laura J. Secord, it is available for $25 from

InterStudy's Center for Aging and Long-Term Care, 5715 Christmas Lake Road, Box 458, Excelsior, MN 55331-0458; (612) 474-1176.

Chore and Homemaker Services

Some older adults are relatively healthy but are unable to carry out a few simple tasks necessary for independent living. These may be as urgent as repairing a burst pipe or as mundane as cleaning the house. Some tasks, such as food shopping, must be performed frequently, while others, such as replacing storm windows with screens, require attention just once or twice a year. Although assistance is available in the community for these and other chores, some older persons do not know where to find help or are reluctant to trust strangers in their homes.

Hospitals can address these needs at relatively little cost and effort. Homemaker, chore, and handyman services can assist older adults with a variety of tasks, including shopping, light cleaning, general errands, and minor home repairs. In addition, a program could offer wake-up and tuck-in services. Some older persons are more likely to feel comfortable with an aide if he or she is affiliated with a hospital-sponsored program.

Most existing programs are relatively small, assisting at most no more than a few dozen clients each week, and often only a handful at one time. Typically, services are provided on a short-term basis, although some clients will need help on an ongoing basis for years.

Homemaker services can be operated through a home health care program, or can be managed separately. Labor costs are low, as aides need little special training and often are paid minimum wage. Some programs are staffed largely or entirely by volunteers. Because no third-party reimbursement is available for these services, clients often pay the hospital a small fee, typically in the range of $3 to $5 per hour. The fee and cost structures allow many homemaker programs to break even on a marginal cost basis.

Promotion and marketing may involve advertisements, newspaper articles, and public service announcements. Hospital discharge planners should be made aware of homemaker programs, since many patients leaving the hospital will be candidates for chore services. As an increasing number of older persons choose to live alone, the need for homemaker services is likely to rise. Such services allow hospitals to discharge some frail older patients earlier than would otherwise be possible, thus saving on care costs. Hospitals also benefit from increased goodwill generated by offering homemaker services.

Financial and Legal Services

Some older adults need assistance with their finances, wills, and insurance policies. A hospital often is in a credible position to supply or recommend these services because of its reputation in the community. Some hospitals provide financial planning services for local elders, either through trained volunteers or through subcontracts with financial planners or institutions. Usually the service is provided at low or no charge. Presumably, many older adults using the service—as well as their families—will think of the sponsoring hospital for their care needs. In addition, some programs have learned information about the financial resources and charitable-giving histories of local elders that have aided their fund-raising campaigns.

Elder legal services often center on assisting older adults in writing wills. Law students or community legal aid societies may supply the counseling expertise free of charge, or may be able to train volunteers to answer basic questions. The sponsoring hospital provides a valuable service and generates goodwill among the local elder community. Other legal issues of particular interest to older persons are living wills, durable powers of attorney, and euthanasia rights.

Some hospitals are starting to offer estate management services to older adults who are moving out of their homes, or to the families of the recently deceased. For example, Huntington Memorial Hospital in Pasadena, California, offers an estate management program affiliated with the hospital gift shop, "The Huntington Collection." The program assesses a situation, appraises assets, packs and moves all items, cleans the home, and, if desired, sells some or all of the property. The service auctions property and receives 35 percent of the funds raised. Furniture and other items appraised at $100 or more are sold on consignment, with the service retaining 35 percent of the sale price. The Huntington Collection provides an important service for older adults moving to other homes or convalescent facilities, and also benefits out-of-town children whose parents have recently died. At the same time, the program raises funds for the hospital. (See Case Study 5 on Huntington Hospital in Chapter 4.)

Information Sources: For more information about The Huntington Collection Estate Management Program, contact The Huntington Collection at 10 Congress Street, Suite 205, Pasadena, CA 91105; (818) 304-9727.

Geriatric Health Assessment

Geriatric health assessment is a valuable health service that will gain in importance as the eldercare system develops. Assessment involves the multidisciplinary evaluation of physical, mental, social, and financial needs, usually for a frail or disabled older adult. Medical diagnosis is one aspect of geriatric health assessment, but the service goes well beyond clinical evaluation to determine what array of services might best serve individuals given their living environment, informal support, and financial resources. Assessment dovetails nicely with case management services to identify needs and arrange care, and this model is likely to become more widespread as the eldercare system expands.

Health assessment may be conducted on either an inpatient or outpatient basis. Inpatient programs are more common; in fact, a large proportion of the nation's dedicated geriatric inpatient programs focus on assessment rather than rehabilitation or general medical care. Some outpatient programs conduct assessments in addition to other services. Many programs are aimed specifically at older persons suffering from dementia. Whatever the arrangement, a complete health assessment procedure typically takes several days to complete.

The process itself involves a full physical exam, a mental status test, a neurological evaluation, and vision and audiological workups. Also included are a psychological interview and an environmental assessment. A variety of professionals usually are involved, including a geriatrician or internist, a neuropsychologist, a clinical pharmacist, a geropsychiatrist, an occupational therapist, a social worker, a registered nurse, and often an audiologist or speech therapist. Besides medical testing and evaluation, the occupational therapist considers the patient's abilities to perform the activities of daily living (ADL) and instrumental activities of daily living (IADL). The social worker assesses the patient's support systems, including family ties, living situation, social environment, and financial resources.

Once the entire assessment is completed, the social worker and program coordinator, who typically is a registered nurse, meet with the family and patient (if appropriate) to discuss the findings and recommendations. Often there will be some follow-up contact a few weeks later. Health assessment usually does not involve arranging for and monitoring care, as these are case management services. On the other hand, case management does involve a health assessment on the front end.

There has been a proliferation of assessment programs in the last five years. Assessment has assumed a pivotal role in geriatric care because of the complexity of the frail elderly patient, the many unmet needs of this growing segment of the population, and the association of assessment with improved outcomes. Extensive reviews of the literature make it clear that assessment programs are effective, practical and important. The evidence indicates that well-run programs can lead to long-term financial savings in the care of the frail elderly by reducing the length of stay in both acute hospitals and nursing homes.

However, growth has been hampered by the lack of any specific provision for special funding under Medicare prospective payment regulations. Medicare provides no financial incentive for the establishment of assessment programs. Nor is there any other adequate funding source. Third-party payers do not yet provide adequate reimbursement. The programs that are most adequately reimbursed are those that function within large prepaid systems, such as the Veterans Administration (VA) and large HMOs.

At present, hospitals can establish assessment programs as part of acute care bed services (with the length of stay determined by DRGs); as part of acute rehabilitation units (though this requires extensive documentation to meet the highly restrictive Medicare guidelines); or by obtaining Medicare waivers as special demonstrations. In the future, we are likely to see the development of cheaper ambulatory facilities (which may be part of a hospital organization, whether or not they are housed in the hospital) and the increased integration of geriatric assessment with the various components of a comprehensive, flexible, community-based long-term care system.

The specific medical goal of health assessment is the identification of patients who are likely to need an even more intensive evaluation, particularly patients who may be in danger of some adverse long-term care episode. Cost effectiveness depends upon careful patient selection.

Health assessment programs generally are not established to earn direct profits. The intensity of professional staff effort needed for an effective program makes it difficult to cover costs, even though most clinicians do not receive the type of compensation for time devoted to assessment services that they do for other procedures. If a diagnosis is reached—which usually happens—Medicare or Medicaid may provide some reimbursement, but this usually is not enough to make a health assessment program self-sustaining. Hospitals offer assessment programs to serve their communities. Hospitals benefit from the goodwill generated and from reimbursement from procedures performed as a result of conditions discovered during the assessment process.

Information Sources: Mount Zion Hospital and Medical Center in San Francisco has a geriatric assessment unit with both inpatient and outpatient components. For more information, contact the Geriatric Assessment Service, Mount Zion Hospital and Medical Center, P.O. Box 7921, San Francisco, CA 94120; (415) 885-7521.

Mount Sinai Medical Center in Milwaukee has an outpatient geriatric assessment program that is incorporated into a number of other leading eldercare services. More information can be obtained through the Geriatrics Institute, Mount Sinai Medical Center, 945 North 12th, Milwaukee, WI; (414) 289-8320.

Durham County General Hospital, 3643 North Roxboro Street, Durham, NC 27705, also has a stellar assessment program as part of its Geriatric Inpatient Unit. Contact the Planning Department at (919) 470-6161.

The February 1987 issue of *Clinic in Geriatric Medicine* is dedicated to assessment, and should be consulted by hospitals considering a program.

Geriatric Inpatient Units

Optimal inpatient treatment for older adults differs from that of younger persons. Because the elderly are at greater risk of losing functional independence, excellent inpatient care often involves motivating patients to strive to regain function. In addition, older persons tend to recover more slowly and less completely than younger persons, often requiring special staff training. Finally, optimal facilities for inpatient eldercare contain unique design elements to compensate for physical and perceptual difficulties and to aid in orientation. For these reasons, some leading eldercare hospitals, including Mount Sinai Medical Center in New York, Mount Zion Hospital and Medical Center in San Francisco, Durham County General Hospital in Durham, North Carolina, and the Robert Wood Johnson University Hospital in New Brunswick, New Jersey, have established dedicated geriatric units.

Currently there are just a handful of geriatric medical inpatient units in the nation, although an increasing number of hospitals are exploring the concept. Somewhat more common are *inpatient geriatric assessment* units, which admit older persons for a few days or a week for evaluative purposes. Also, there are several hundred *inpatient geriatric rehabilitation* programs in America.

A *geriatric medical inpatient unit* better serves the care needs of certain older patients. The hospital benefits by focusing its elder inpatient resources in one unit, which is advantageous from both operations and marketing standpoints. An institution with a designated unit for older adults positions itself as caring about the elderly and having particular expertise in geriatric medicine.

Costs for establishing a geriatric inpatient unit are relatively minor; often the unit will be a portion of a larger medical-surgical section or floor. Start-up expenses may include carpeting, railings, repainting, clocks, modified furniture, and so forth. The only actual structural renovation that may be necessary involves rearranging walls and doors to expand some private rooms into semiprivate or four-bed rooms, since socialization can be instrumental in recovery for disoriented older persons. (The first section of this chapter details many of the design characteristics that meet the needs of older adults.)

Revenue sources, unit management, and staffing ratios are similar to those of other inpatient units, meaning that little new managerial expertise is required to open a geriatric inpatient unit. However, there are some differences in unit operation. Special admitting criteria may be established and communicated to physicians to ensure proper use of the unit. These might include a minimum age (perhaps 70 or 75), rehabilitation potential, and some capacity for self-care or family care. Physical, speech, occupational, and recreational therapists might visit the floor instead of the patients traveling to a special area within the hospital. Staff sensitivity training to the special needs of older adults is important.

Costs also may differ for a geriatric inpatient unit, although the lack of data makes generalization difficult. Durham County General Hospital in Durham, North Carolina, established a 39-bed geriatric care unit in 1984 with grant funding. It now operates as part of the hospital without special funding. In comparison to a similar, nongeriatric medical unit used as a control, operating costs for the special unit have been higher during some months, but lower at other times. The geriatric unit generally has more nursing hours per patient but less use of ancillary services. Most of the care is primary, and emphasis is placed on continuity of care between each patient and a particular staff member or members, using multidisciplinary teams and a nurse-to-patient ratio of one to four during the day and one to five or six at night.

The hospital also compared the medical outcomes, and the financial results, of the geriatric unit to a control unit that did not provide medical assessments or primary care nursing. The medical outcomes were definitely better in the geriatric unit, where parents showed increased functional capacity and improved mental states. The financial news varied with the diagnosis. Some diagnoses, such as pneumonia or gastrointestinal illness, showed better cost-benefit ratios in the geriatric unit. Others, such as cerebral vascular disease, did not.

Information Sources: For further information, contact the Director of Planning, Durham County General Hospital, 3643 North Roxboro Street, Durham, NC 27705; (919) 470-6161.

Another geriatric inpatient unit was recently implemented at the Robert Wood Johnson University Hospital, 1 Robert Wood Johnson Plaza, New Brunswick, NJ 08901; (201) 937-8607.

Health Promotion and Wellness

Health promotion is a general term describing a spectrum of activities designed to foster optimal health and wellness. These activities aim to increase awareness of factors affecting health and to influence behavior toward functional independence and overall well being. The health promotion field encompasses various types of education, wellness activities, and preventive measures, and usually is offered to complement more traditional acute medical activities.

Health promotion education is intended to promote understanding of factors affecting health, to teach individuals to maintain or improve their health, and to train individuals in the use of emergency procedures, such as cardiopulmonary resuscitation (CPR) or first aid. Education can be fostered by offering ongoing health classes, special presentations, fairs, and workshops, or by establishing a community aging resource center. Wellness activities usually are interactive and typically are designed to increase fitness (through exercise programs), enhance nutrition (through meals served in congregate settings or delivered to homes), maintain involvement with others (through social or recreational programs, such as peer support groups), or stimulate mental faculties (through activities requiring participation and response, such as behavior change workshops). Preventive measures aim to detect health problems before they become serious (through screening programs), establish procedures for dealing with emergencies (such as emergency response systems), or encourage individuals to lead healthier life-styles (for example, with stress management, smoking cessation, or weight loss programs). In a sense, all health promotion activities are preventive, since all are intended to prevent the occurrence or exacerbation of illness.

In practice, health promotion is a broad field involving a variety of types of activities. Most hospital-based programs include some but not all of these services and may organize services under one or more departments. From a planning perspective, it is useful to separate activities by provider and point of delivery. Under these distinctions, educational and programmatic activities, such as self-care lectures or fitness classes, differ from procedural or administrative activities, such as health screening, congregate meals, or emergency medical response systems. Here we will focus on developing a health promotion program involving the former group of services, which tend to require similar or coordinated planning. Other sections discuss design and implementation of services more individual in their management requirements.

Specifically, a health promotion program may include some or all of the following:

- *health education classes*, focusing on preventing disease, reducing the risk of illness, or coping with chronic conditions;

- *self-care instruction*, including proper use of the health care system, self-monitoring, and safe use of medication;

- *accident prevention counseling*, emphasizing awareness of risk factors and encouraging such preventive measures as seat-belt use and home safety modification;

- *healthy living classes and workshops*, describing stress reduction techniques and providing life planning, nutritional, and other useful life-style information;

- *behavior change programs*, such as smoking cessation, weight loss, and stress reduction;

- *peer support groups*, such as grief, loss, Alzheimer's, and coping-with-illness programs;

- *emergency medical training*, such as CPR and first aid;

- *physical fitness and exercise programs;* and
- *life enhancement programs,* providing opportunities for socializing and deeper involvement with society.

Traditionally, health promotion programs have focused on the young, who were considered to have the most to gain from such services, at least in terms of years. However, as life expectancy has increased and as a growing body of research has documented the value of health improvement services to older persons, the health promotion field has expanded to include the elderly. A major survey of community hospitals by the American Hospital Association found that over 60 percent of respondents offer some type of elder health promotion services, although just 3.3 percent have programs specifically designed for older adults. Elderly needs may be different from those of younger persons, but the benefits of health promotion are no less important.

Value: Health promotion programs for the elderly are intended to improve health and well being, primarily through nonmedical techniques. The ultimate goal is to make wellness a natural part of living. Benefits to the elderly include better physical and mental health, an enhanced feeling of well-being, a sense of purpose, opportunities for socializing and recreation, and a wiser, more efficient use of medical services.

Hospitals offer health promotion services for a number of reasons. Such services tend to further the organizational goal of improving community health and providing optimal service to the elderly. A good health promotion program can be an excellent marketing and public relations tool, increasing a hospital's visibility and contributing to its image as a progressive, health-oriented institution. Also, health promotion activities often act as feeders for traditional hospital services. These programs represent one of the most effective ways of attracting relatively healthy older individuals to a hospital.

Financially, health promotion services are rarely sponsored to earn a profit. Some programs are established with the goal of breaking even, while others expect that costs will exceed revenues, sometimes by a substantial amount. Hospitals often sponsor health promotion programs as loss-leaders for other services. However, health promotion programs can reap significant benefits for a hospital without requiring large investments of money or staff time. For example, North Country Hospital in Newport, Vermont, established a senior health promotion program with an initial investment of $13,500; in 1985, revenues exceeded direct costs.

Cost: Because the scope, depth, and intensity of health promotion programs vary greatly, costs range from very little to hundreds of thousands of dollars. A modest program may require no capital investments whatsoever, since most facilities and equipment either will be available within the hospital or may be borrowed from other organizations. One-time development costs also may be minimal, primarily involving a needs assessment survey and initial marketing expenses. Excellent hospital-based health promotion programs have been established for under $20,000. The American Hospital Association recently sponsored a teleconference describing effective health promotion ideas for older adults for under $5000.

Volunteers can be used to minimize program costs. These may include individuals from the hospital volunteer organization who are trained to provide health promotion services as well as experts from the hospital staff and the community. In addition, local organizations may donate staff, facilities, materials, and services, and often are willing to cosponsor the entire program. This both defrays costs and reduces the need for staff time.

Staffing: The nature, form, and scope of a health promotion program will determine its staffing needs. Most programs will have a paid coordinator or administrator with a background in nursing, health education, public health, or administration. There usually is a training and support staff. Smaller programs may have just one or two paid FTEs and usually several part-time employees.

Volunteers account for the majority of most health promotion staffs. They may serve as patient education coordinators, perform administrative tasks, and provide transportation or telephone reassurance services. A primary task of the program administrator is volunteer recruitment and supervision.

Hospital staff, such as nurses, physicians, and social workers, may be used as speakers for programs. Fitness instructors, psychologists, nutritionists, and health lecturers may be hired from the local community resource pool on a per-course basis, thus limiting program fixed costs. Community organizations such as the Red Cross, the American Cancer Society, the People's Council on Physical Fitness, or the local rescue squad may be eager to provide educators or other sources of staff support.

Revenues: The typical health promotion program receives revenues from multiple sources. Although few preventive health services are reimbursed by public or private payers, some classes can be designed to take advantage of policies covering patient education essential to care. For the most part, however, revenues must come from other sources.

Health promotion programs typically receive most of their funding from the sponsoring hospital. Additionally, hospitals often cover such indirect costs as site, utilities, telephone, and office expenses. Because health promotion specifically oriented toward the elderly is not yet widespread, many programs have been successful in getting grants to fund start-up expenditures. For example, the elder health promotion program at Illinois Masonic Medical Center in Chicago received nearly 30 percent of its funding from a locally based national foundation. Grants typically come from the federal, state, or local government. Foundations are another source of grant money, although access to smaller foundations may be difficult. Hospital foundations often find senior health promotion programs appealing; Foothill Presbyterian Hospital in Glendora, California, funds nearly 40 percent of its program through the hospital's Health and Education Foundation.

Corporations may provide financial assistance through either cash or in-kind donations. Local businesses, especially retailers, may be willing to support a program as a goodwill or promotional gesture. Often in-kind donations are made more generously than cash contributions.

Finally, an increasing number of hospital-based programs charge fees for health promotion services. The fee component varies from 5 to 50 percent of expenses, most typically falling in the 15 to 25 percent range. Fees for programs rarely exceed $20 and often are requested as donations.

Market: Given the varied nature of health promotion services, a broad view of the market includes nearly all older persons living in the community and, possibly, even some in institutions. Programs for older adults may be aimed not only at the elderly but at all persons over age 50 or 55. Of course, an effective health promotion program will focus on particular segments of the local market and design services to address that population's needs. Targeted segments might include the well elderly, the frail elderly, children and families of the elderly, and centralized retirement communities.

Typically, health promotion programs will cater to reasonably healthy elderly persons living in their own homes. Although many of these individuals suffer from chronic conditions, most are ambulatory and able to care for themselves independently. Some hospital-based health promotion programs are expanding in order to serve the disabled elderly population and those involved with home care services.

Marketing: Successful health promotion programs tend to emphasize the aspect of marketing that many hospitals neglect: consumer-driven program design. Initial market research, usually in the form of a basic needs assessment survey, is crucial. The survey should attempt to determine potential topics of interest, as well as preferred format, time, and location. If possible, a pilot class or service should be offered to test the program concept. Many sponsors find it useful to repeat the market survey on a regular basis, often biannually.

A variety of methods for recruiting participants is available. Print advertising is one of the most common; newsletters for hospitals, churches, and senior centers are ideal, as are articles or ads in local newspapers. Radio and cable television spots may also yield results. Other possibilities include flyers, brochures, posters, and telephone advertising. Some programs have gone even further, offering balloons, shoelaces, toothbrushes, and chicken soup. Many health promotion programs cite word of mouth advertising as their most successful promotional tool, albeit the one over which they have the least control.

Providers are an important part of the health promotion market. Physicians, nurses, physical and occupational therapists, and other providers are all potential referral sources and possible speakers. Some health promotion programs have used creative methods to tie in these providers. One example is "prescription forms" that the health promotion programs distribute to providers. The health professionals then can "write a prescription" for health and wellness classes for their patients. At the very least, physicians should be made aware of the various health promotion services available for older patients.

Other means of marketing health promotion programs for the elderly include offering college credits for courses, providing transportation to and from programs, and linking classes with social or recreational events. Cosponsoring events with senior groups, such as the local senior center or AARP chapter, is another way to market a health promotion program.

Competition: As health promotion programs directed at the elderly increase in number, hospitals will find themselves competing with one another for participants. Presently, however, most such programs are offered by not-for-profit community organizations such as the Red Cross, the American Heart Association, the American Cancer Society, or the local area agency on aging. These groups may turn out to be hospital allies rather than competitors. Since health promotion programs rarely make money and usually cost much more than they collect in fees, many not-for-profit organizations are willing to share the financial burden with hospitals. Joint-venturing with such a group allows a hospital to gain experience while saving money.

If another local hospital sponsors a health promotion program, it may or may not represent competition. The range of potential services is wide enough so that many programs could be offered without redundancy. Another option is to collaborate with the competing hospital; the greater efficiency and lower costs of such an arrangement must be weighed against the division of the referrals from the program between the two institutions.

Timetable: The time required to establish a health promotion program depends largely on the nature, number, and scope of services offered. Modest programs beginning with only a few health education courses can be started in a matter of weeks, if necessary. However, programs designed to serve a strategic function within a hospital's eldercare effort will require more development time.

A meaningful needs assessment is likely to take at least one or two months and sometimes much longer, including the time needed to meet with community groups. Fund-raising, hiring of staff, program development, and a basic marketing campaign may take from several months to two years. Most good hospital-based health promotion programs are developed over a period of at least a year, and it is not at all unusual for several years to elapse between initial conception and the provision of a fully integrated spectrum of services. The time frame often is extended because development staff may not be working on the project full time.

Management: Most hospital-based health promotion programs are either managed entirely by hospital staff or joint ventured with community organizations. Which avenue a hospital should select depends on available resources, program goals and scope, and existing local programs. If successful community programs exist, collaboration allows a hospital to shorten or eliminate the needs analysis, fund-raising, and premarketing processes. The hospital can contribute institutional resources, marketing expertise, meeting facilities, transportation, and its reputation to the program.

Ambitious health promotion programs tend to be hospital-managed. This does not preclude cosponsorship of individual services with other organizations. However, it increases the likelihood that the program will best meet the needs of both the elderly population and the hospital. Responsibilities for health promotion services for older adults typically are based in the health promotion, education, social service, public relations, or geriatrics departments. Traditionally, the program administrator may coordinate all senior services or may have responsibility for health promotion activities for all age groups.

As hospitals reorganize and develop increasingly complex corporate structures, some institutions are separately incorporating divisions that provide health promotion and wellness services. The rationale for such restructuring involves improved financial and administrative flexibility. Managerial issues are similar to those of programs operated from within a traditional hospital organization.

Development Concerns: Health promotion services for the elderly may be incorporated into existing programs. Health education can be included in an adult day care or home health care program, nutrition education can be a component of a congregate meals program, and instructions in proper use of the health care system can be a part of a case management program. This combining of services enhances the care continuum offered by hospitals to the elderly.

The initial needs assessment should include older adults and representatives from agencies and community organizations serving the elderly. A broad questionnaire or survey is also useful for determining the target market's needs and preferences. Program location and timing, as well as transportation needs, are key determinants of success. Once the program is under way, subsequent evaluations and refinements should involve participants.

Hospitals concerned about minimizing financial outlays should design services for maximum subsidization. Because many patient education services associated with medical treatment are reimbursed, these educational services can be emphasized and marketed to potential consumers as a no-cost benefit. Similarly, programs can be developed that are likely to interest corporations or foundations, increasing the likelihood of grants, donations, or subsidies from those sources.

Information Sources: Perhaps the best source of information about hospital-based health promotion programs is the Center for Health Promotion of the American Hospital Association, 840 North Lake Shore Drive, Chicago, IL 60611; (312) 280-6000. The Center has several publications on health promotion and wellness, as well as teleconferences featuring program managers from several hospitals.

Another source is the Health Advocacy department of the American Association of Retired Persons, 1909 K Street, N.W., Washington, DC 20049; (202) 728-4450.

The Healthy Older People program at the Department of Health and Human Services is another excellent source of information. The address is 801 North Capitol Street, N.E., Washington, DC 20002; (202) 245-7611.

Wellness and Health Promotion for the Elderly, edited by Ken Dychtwald (Aspen Systems Corporation, Rockville, Maryland, 1986) provides a wealth of medical, descriptive, and planning information about health promotion, as well as case studies of community and hospital-based programs. Aspen's phone number is (301) 251-5000.

Health Screening

The elderly are at greater risk than younger age groups for chronic health problems. However, the misperception that deteriorating health is a natural and inevitable concomitant of aging leads to a high degree of unrecognized medical conditions in the elderly. Many of these problems could be prevented, arrested, postponed, or minimized with early diagnosis and treatment. Health screening programs offered to the elderly can detect potential or existing conditions before they become serious health risks.

Screening usually focuses on four types of problems:

1. *physical conditions,* such as glaucoma, hypertension, certain cancers, hearing disorders, and diabetes. Because the elderly are at greater risk for these conditions than are younger persons, screening can be particularly useful in detecting problems early.

2. *mental disorders,* including depression and senile dementia. Approximately half of the senile dementias and many cases of depression can be reversed or controlled if diagnosed early enough.

3. *nutritional deficiencies,* which often cause or exacerbate other health problems. Undernourishment can result from a lack of mealtime companions, side effects of pharmaceuticals on nutrient absorption, or a loss of taste buds leading to lack of appetite.

4. *drugs and drug interactions,* which often lead to problems among the elderly population. Older adults use nearly a third of all prescription drugs in this country, and up to one-fourth of hospital admissions of the elderly result from drug reactions or interactions.

Health screening services may be provided at a hospital, a designated health center, a senior center or retirement community, a shopping mall, or elsewhere. A program may offer just one service, such as hypertension screening, or a broad spectrum, as within the context of a health fair. Some programs remain open on a regular basis, perhaps 40 hours per week, while others are offered at distinct intervals, perhaps monthly or biweekly.

Value: Health screening benefits the elderly by detecting potential problems before they become serious. Many conditions can be reversed if recognized early enough. Health screening also allows older persons to receive (at no or low cost in a convenient setting) diagnostic services and information about possible treatment.

Hospitals offer health screening services for several reasons. Such programs tend to further the organizational mission of improving community health. They represent excellent public relations vehicles. Health screening programs provide hospitals with opportunities to establish or strengthen ties with community organizations serving the elderly, as well as with older persons themselves. Finally, health screening programs can generate referrals, providing a natural entry point into a hospital's elder service network. It is not uncommon for 25 to 50 percent of older persons tested to be found to have significant health problems, often requiring treatment and referral. Because those needing treatment are more likely than others to lack a personal physician, a health screening program sometimes can refer patients in need to doctors affiliated with the sponsoring hospital.

While health screening programs may generate some revenues, rarely do they earn significant direct profits. However, referrals resulting from health problems detected through certain screening programs can be quite profitable. Depending on the volume and types of referrals likely to be generated, a typical screening program can result in profits ranging from a few thousand to tens of thousands of dollars annually for the hospital and physicians involved.

Cost: The cost of a health screening program depends on its scope, site, and staff. The breadth of services offered has a large impact on costs, since certain procedures require relatively sophisticated equipment while others, such as vision screening, can be performed with simple materials. Some services must involve physicians or experienced technicians, while others can use trained laypersons.

For a program offered at regular intervals—as opposed to a service available on a daily basis—it is not uncommon to spend from $500 to $700 per screening in marketing expenses. Set-up and administrative costs for a one-day eye screening of approximately 40 individuals can run another $500. An ongoing service will have higher overhead costs, although marketing expenses may be similar.

Several steps can be taken to minimize operating costs. Smaller programs may save on marketing costs by relying on physician referrals and word of mouth. Locating a health screening program in a hospital can reduce the expense of moving equipment and staff to another site. Using hospital or community facilities may eliminate rental costs, although major health fairs may require renting a convention hall or other large space. Another way to minimize costs is to make extensive use of volunteers, who can be trained to measure blood pressure and assist with other procedures.

An excellent means of minimizing operating costs is to use community organizations, such as the Red Cross and American Cancer Society, to conduct the screenings. This has the additional advantage of building bridges with the local aging network.

Staffing: Many health screening programs will use one or more physician(s), depending on the size of the service and the number of health parameters being tested. For example, a one-day health screening program that tests 40 older adults will require at least one physician, an assistant, and three or four helpers. However, a bare-bones program could get by with one physician, an assistant, and a helper. Some screenings do not require direct physician involvement; many make use of lay professionals.

In some programs, physicians are not paid for their screening services. Their primary incentive is the referrals that the program generates, of which there can be many, particularly for a service such as glaucoma screening. In some cases, even a physician who accepts Medicare assignment and waives coinsurance for resulting procedures probably will benefit from donating his or her services to a health screening program.

For some types of procedures, it is important that the assistant has clinical or technical training. Other procedures can substitute trained volunteers. The helpers generally need no special training, but are present to prepare participants and arrange for their subsequent needs, if any. In order to make best use of clinicians' time during a health fair, the helpers must make certain that there is always a person available for the physician to screen without needless time lags between procedures. After the screening is completed, the helpers arrange follow-up appointments if necessary.

Revenues: A health screening program may or may not generate substantial revenues from direct services, depending on the nature of the program. The majority of screening programs provide their services free of charge. However, others charge from $30 to $50 for a screening, which can generate several thousand dollars per month in revenue and allow an ongoing program to break even. Medicare and private insurance generally do not cover screening services, although reimbursement is occasionally available if the procedure is recommended by a physician.

It is possible that local businesses, particularly those that sell to the elderly or their families, might contribute funds to sponsor health screenings, especially within the context of a large health fair. In return for a $200 or $500 sponsorship, a corporation would have its name prominently displayed on all promotional materials. Sponsorship levels need not be correlated with direct costs, since sponsors are paying for the positive publicity; in other words, the fee is more a marketing expense than a charitable contribution. Several local businesses that do not compete with one another might each sponsor a portion of a health fair. Many older persons greatly appreciate free services, handouts, and gifts, and screening sponsors that provide such items can reap significant public relations benefits.

Beyond the direct revenues raised by the screening itself, a health screening program can be financially beneficial due to the referrals it might generate. For certain types of screening, these revenues and their associated profits can be significant. For example, ElderMed, which sells a packaged eye care screening program for hospitals, estimates that about 10 percent of older adults screened will need and undergo cataract surgery. If 40 persons per month are screened, approximately 48 operations will be performed per year as a result, generating perhaps from $40,000 to $60,000 in net revenues and from $30,000 to $40,000 in gross profits for the hospital and physicians involved. Other types of screening programs may be likely to result in somewhat less revenue, but can nonetheless be financially worthwhile.

Market: Screening is most beneficial to both the community and the hospital when those tested have the greatest likelihood of suffering from undiagnosed ailments. This population will tend to be older, although age is only a very rough indicator of health risk. These individuals probably have not seen a physician or been hospitalized recently, unless they are referred to a health screening clinic by a professional. The geographic market for health screening extends throughout a hospital's service area and perhaps somewhat beyond.

Other markets for health screening services include the families of the elderly, elder organizations, senior centers, and local providers. The hospital medical staff should be happy to recommend the program and display promotional materials in their offices, although it is likely that older adults who visit physicians are slightly less in need of many screening services than are other older persons who do not visit a physician regularly.

Marketing: Many candidates for health screening might be found in nursing homes, retirement communities, life care centers, or senior housing. Residents generally are over age 60, and on average may be somewhat less healthy than older adults living fully independently. These concentrated older populations facilitate marketing efforts: not only can they be reached efficiently through announcements at central locations, but the screening itself can be held on site. Some hospitals sponsor mobile units with staffs of two or three to administer tests at various locations. Another option is to provide transportation to and from health screenings for older adults living in specialized settings.

Direct mail is another means of promoting health screening services. An excellent list to use is the membership roster of a hospital's senior access program. Other mailing lists of older adults can be purchased from local brokers. Additional mailings should be sent to elder organizations and senior centers, perhaps with posters for display. Radio spots also can be useful promotional vehicles and may be broadcast free as public service announcements.

Physicians can be the single most important referral source for a screening program. Some physicians routinely require their patients to undergo certain types of health screening as part of a standard check-up. However, many doctors are unfamiliar with the specifics of the process and consider screening a poor way to diagnose health problems. A program that is marketed to physicians as a screening service leading to further testing, rather than a diagnostic instrument whose results are clear-cut, is more likely to be accepted and recommended by physicians.

Pricing can be an issue for health screening programs. The majority of hospital-based programs offer free screening services. Although this may forego some direct revenues, it also avoids a potential barrier to participation. If charging for health screening reduces participation to any significant extent, the sponsoring hospital will lose far more in referral revenues than it will gain in direct fees.

However, many older adults are quite willing to pay for certain types of screening. Market research can help determine how a screening service should be priced. After an extensive market survey, Baptist Medical Center in Oklahoma City set its osteoporosis screening fee at $405, and typically sees from 30 to 40 patients per month in its clinic.

Competition: Competition for health screening services will come from other hospitals, community organizations such as the Red Cross, and local physicians. The most significant competitors may be other hospitals. Organizations and physicians may be willing to collaborate with hospitals to offer health screening services, since a hospital's reputation, financial resources, marketing channels, and physical facilities can be important assets in providing services.

A typical hospital will find a number of health screening programs offered within its service area. However, there is a wide variety of screening services that can be offered, and few programs offer most or all of them. Therefore, a program can be designed to fit a market niche in which there is little competition. The disadvantage of this strategy is that some of the occupied niches may be among the most profitable.

Timetable: A health screening program can be planned and initiated in a short period of time. A simple screening involving just one type of test—for example, hearing—can be conceived, marketed, and offered within a few months. A prepackaged program, such as any of the several sold by ElderMed, can be operational within a month. Most of the lead time needed is used for reserving a site and marketing the program.

An ongoing program sited within a hospital may take slightly longer to establish, depending on the degree of renovation required. Nevertheless, the hiring of staff, purchasing of equipment, and structural modification usually can all be completed within six months.

Management: A health screening program does not require extensive management resources and might be coordinated by any of a number of different departments. Hospitals often assign responsibility for overseeing elder health screening programs to the manager of eldercare services, if someone has been so designated. Otherwise, leadership may rest with nursing or patient care services or with the marketing department. The ideal leader will have excellent community contacts and organizing skills.

Development Concerns: Market research may be required to determine what types of screening are already available in the community and what services are needed. A hospital should think carefully before entering into competition with community-based providers, to avoid both duplicating services and competing with potential allies. Community agencies may make ideal joint-venture partners for offering health screening programs.

Site location is another important issue. Although there are some advantages to offering screening services within the hospital, the majority of programs are held in the community. Some hospitals have mobile screening units—usually housed in large trailers—that travel to churches, senior centers, shopping malls, or other places where elders congregate. Whatever the site, access to transportation is critical for a successful program.

The medical staff should be involved in the design and implementation of a health screening program. Private attending physicians sometimes criticize health fairs for the impersonal, assembly line system used to test a large number of elders in a short period of time. Physician support may be gained by inviting the medical staff to participate (when the nature of screening requires medical training) and by incorporating a referral service into the program.

Information Sources: ElderMed sells prepackaged health screening programs to members and nonmembers. Contact ElderMed at 20500 Nordhoff Street, Chatsworth, CA 91311; (818) 407-2207.

Home Health Care

The home health care industry is burgeoning, but the details of that growth have changed radically in the last few years. While many new ventures are arising, many others are folding. Hospital-based programs continue to grow, as does the number of private-pay patients, but the rate of growth of the Medicare-funded segment has dropped seriously.

Spurred by increases in both public and private funds, expenditures for home health care increased at an average annual rate of 31 percent during the 1970s and the early 1980s. About 40 to 42 million home health visits were provided in the United States during 1988, up from only 6 million in 1970, according to the National Association of Home Care (NAHC). The Congressional Budget Office estimates that expenditures reached $9.1 billion in 1985; market researcher Frost and Sullivan, Inc., expects that figure to reach $16 billion by 1990. About 70 percent of the total is for services. More than half of it is paid for privately, 80 percent of that out-of-pocket.

The total number of agencies nationwide was estimated by the NAHC to have reached 12,000 by April 1988. The majority of these agencies are freestanding and provide private-pay but not Medicare services. Almost all hospital-based programs offer Medicare services, and increasing numbers are expanding into the private-pay market. In 1984, just over 40 percent of the nation's hospitals offered home health care services; by 1985, the proportion had risen to nearly two-thirds.

Looking at just the Medicare part of the market gives a different picture. The number of Medicare-certified home health agencies soared from 1465 in 1970, to 2858 in 1979, 5237 in 1984, and 6007 in 1986. Medicare expenditures on home health grew from $1.4 billion in 1983 to an estimated $2.6 billion in 1988 and a projected $3 billion by 1990. But what is equally interesting is the change in the rate of growth. From yearly increases in excess of 30 percent before prospective payment system (PPS) legislation, the rate of growth dropped in 1985 to 14.1 percent, in 1986 to 4.7 percent, and in 1988 to an estimated 2.8 percent. From its 1986 high of 6007, the number of Medicare-certified agencies dropped to 5787 in 1988— 695 new agencies started, but 915 closed. Almost all of the increase in funding these days is due to the inflation of costs per visit. In the face of a soaring population of frail elderly, there is very little growth in the number of Medicare-sponsored visits to their homes.

Perhaps more important, all of the Medicare provisions, even those in the new catastrophic legislation, are based on the image of an acute disease. Medicare is restricted to care that is "intermittent." No provision is made to help people with chronic problems avoid the acute episodes that would put them in the hospital.

Besides the tightening of Medicare reimbursement policies, there are two other factors that have influenced the industry greatly in the last few years. The first is simply that people have become more familiar with home health services, and more ready to make use of them. The second is a direct result of DRGs: people are coming home sooner and sicker, with a much greater need for home health services, for much more intensive services, for more equipment [such as respirators and intravenous (IV) equipment], and for a higher level of skill.

According to research by the Institute for Health and Aging at the University of California at San Francisco, since the PPS legislation, 72 percent of agencies report an increased workload, over half have added fees or copayments, almost half have added services (such as IV therapy), 68 percent have more clients, and 80 percent say their clients are sicker.

Home health care consists of services and products designed to help individuals remain in the community and to compensate for their loss of function. Services may be medical, social, or supportive; this section addresses only the former. Medical services may be skilled or unskilled. Skilled medical services include physician care, skilled nursing care, health assessment, individual and family counseling, home chemotherapy, and physical, speech, and occupational therapy. These may also include providing health or nutrition information to a homebound person or training a patient how to use high-tech medical equipment in the home. Unskilled medical services include custodial care, assistance with basic activities, meal preparation, and transportation to and from the hospital.

Home health care products may be high or low tech. High-tech products include home infusion therapy products and pharmaceuticals. Low-tech products include consumables, such as bandages, and durable medical equipment (DME), such as crutches and wheel-chairs.

Value: Home care boasts many advantages. Most people prefer it to institutionalization. Treating a patient at home maintains personal dignity and family integrity. Since the formal provider usually supplements care that is given by a relative or friend, the combined care efforts actually may be greater than those received by institutionalized patients. Because home care, as opposed to hospital or nursing home care, involves a familiar environment, the patient may actually recover faster.

The hospital also receives benefits from providing home health care services. The program is a feeder for acute care services. Home health care departments also serve as marketing tools by bringing a hospital representative into the community. Finally, home health care decreases a hospital's exposure to malpractice suits for early discharge under PPS.

In addition to marketing, referral, and risk benefits, home health care also may be financially rewarding. Hospital-based home health care allows institutions to continue to draw revenue from discharged patients, an increasingly important consideration with the growth of prospective reimbursement. Medicare reimburses only for costs incurred, but a properly structured home health care agency will allow hospital overhead costs to be spread over a broader base. In fact, the benefits of allocating existing overhead often are greater than the excess of revenues over costs: 25 to 40 percent of the average hospital-sponsored home health care agency budget consists of existing hospital overhead allocated to the agency. Table 3-2 illustrates how a typical hospital-based home health agency can offset existing hospital overhead.

Medicaid reimburses on a fee-for-service basis, allowing a small profit at best. However, the burgeoning private-pay market can be reasonably profitable, depending on local market conditions. At present, programs such as durable medical equipment, home infusion therapy, self-care, and wellness tend to be quite profitable for many agencies. However, prospective payment and increased regulation on the one hand and growing competition on the other threaten to make all aspects of the home care business more challenging in the future.

TABLE 3-2
Hospital-Based Home Health Service: Offsetting Existing Overhead

Resource	Before home health*	With home health services	
		Hospital	Home health†
Senior RN	$ 25,000	$ —	$25,000
Staff RN	20,000	10,000	10,000
Physical therapist	25,000	12,500	12,500
Occupational therapist	21,000	14,000	7,000
Speech therapist	21,000	14,000	7,000
Nutritionist	20,000	15,000	5,000
Receptionist	12,000	6,000	6,000
Office space at $1/ft²/month, 1000 ft²	12,000		12,000
Equipment and furniture	2,000		2,000
Maintenance utilities	2,800		2,800
Telephone line	1,200		1,200
	$162,000	$71,500	$90,500

*Assumes existing resources with excess capacity.
†Reimbursed by Medicare Part A.
Source: Evashwick and Read, 1984

Cost: Actual capital expenditures for establishing a hospital-based home health care organization tend to be minimal: a Federal Trade Commission (FTC) study found that the capital costs required to establish a home health care agency averaged about $15,000. However, the funds needed to capitalize a home care business, including equipment, salaries, and the first several months of receivables, are significant. A hospital with a sizable home health care service program might spend $500,000 to $750,000 financing the venture.

An agency offering home care products will have substantially higher capital expenditures due to investments in inventory. A small but increasing number of hospital-based home care programs offer high-tech equipment. A larger proportion rent, lease, or sell DME. Over half of discharged Medicare patients use DME at home; the average duration of use is about six months, with expenses of approximately $100 month. The share of home health care expenditures consumed by DME and supplies (as opposed to services) is projected to rise from 30 or 40 percent to nearly 50 percent by the year 2000. Many hospitals do not operate their own DME program, but subcontract to an existing firm; a typical subcontract margin would be 35 percent.

Staffing: Home health care medical services more often involve an unskilled attendant than a skilled nurse. Of visits requiring skilled care, between two-thirds and three-fourths will require an RN, with the rest involving a licensed vocational nurse (LVN). Relatively few physicians are directly involved in home care visits, largely because their time is too expensive for either publicly or privately financed visits. Although Medicare requires physicians to supervise home health care treatment plans, their involvement is usually limited to approving the plans of others.

While some agencies keep nurses on staff, an increasing number have adopted an independent practice model in which nurses are paid on a per-visit basis. This allows the agency to pay no more staff than is warranted by demand for services. A nurse can average over six visits per day. In addition to the general clinical staff, a home health care program will require an administrator, a nursing coordinator, and a small support staff.

Revenues: An aggressive hospital-based home health services program can generate $1 million to $2 million in annual revenues. Activities such as DME and infusion therapy can raise revenues far higher. A typical hospital-based agency might have 80 percent of revenues generated by Medicare, 5 to 10 percent from private-pay patients, and the remainder from other sources, including health maintenance organizations. The other source category is growing, as private insurers increasingly cover home health care as an alternative to inpatient care. Nine of ten Blue Cross and Blue Shield plans and about half of commercial insurance policies cover home care, although there are restrictions on the type and duration of coverage.

Medicare began providing expanded home care medical coverage in 1982, including part-time skilled nursing care, physical therapy, or speech therapy. These services must be rendered in accordance with a physician's treatment plan, although direct physician participation may be, and usually is, minimal. The patient must be homebound to be eligible for Medicare reimbursement. Once qualified on the above basis, the patient is eligible for ancillary services, including occupational therapy, home health aides, medical supplies (except outpatient drugs), and DME rental. Most of these services are limited in duration—usually two to four months, subject to renewal every 60 days—and are not intended to substitute for long-term care. There is no deductible for Medicare home care services. Most private insurers use these guidelines in defining their home health care policies.

Current Medicare reimbursement rates for home health care services average about $50 per visit, but vary widely along four dimensions: the nature of service provided, the urban or rural character of the region, the agency's affiliation (or lack of affiliation) with a hospital, and the area's hospital wage index rate. The upper limits of reimbursement for skilled nursing, physical therapy, speech pathology, occupational therapy, and medical social services are from 5 to 10 percent higher for home care agencies outside of metropolitan statistical areas (MSAs); limits for home health aides are slightly higher for agencies within MSAs. Hospital-based programs receive an add-on of approximately 11 percent. The wage index, which may vary as much as 40 percent from the mean, is used to adjust the labor component of the visit, which accounts for the bulk of the charge. Medicare requires extensive documentation and retroactively denies reimbursement for a portion of claims.

Medicaid also finances some amount of home health care services. Federal Medicaid guidelines require states to provide skilled nursing care and home health aide services. Other services are optional, and about a third of all states cover some personal and housekeeping services if they are related to a medical need. Services must be ordered by a physician and supervised by a licensed nurse. States vary widely in their use of Medicaid to fund home health care: in 1980, for example, New York accounted for 40 percent of the nation's recipients, half of Medicaid home health care expenditures, and 90 percent of Medicaid personal care expenditures. Low Medicaid reimbursement rates relative to Medicare rates probably discourage many providers from serving Medicaid recipients, although hospital-based home health care agencies in many states are able to make a small profit from Medicaid patients.

The private-pay market is the most lucrative of home care markets, despite its lower charges than Medicare. No documentation is required, and thus a private-pay program has much lower overhead costs than a Medicare program. Medicare drives the private-pay market, since a majority of private-pay patients are former Medicare patients who no longer meet the strict eligibility requirements. As Medicare has become more stringent in reimbursement, the private-pay segment of the market has grown—by 1988 it represented half of the average agency's load.

Market: The elderly account for between 75 and 90 percent of all home health care services provided. A recent study by Liu et al., based on the 1982 long-term care survey, found that the disabled elderly population living in the community had the following characteristics: 35 percent male, 42 percent married, 15 percent on Medicaid, with a median age of 76 and median family income of $8500. In terms of the market for home care services, just over one-fourth of this group were assisted by paid caregivers either solely or in conjunction with nonpaid caregivers. Relative to the entire disabled elderly population, those with paid caregivers were older, less likely to be male or married or on Medicaid, and more than twice as wealthy (as measured by median family income). Those paying $136 or more per month out of pocket for home care had a median age of 81 and a median family income of $13,000; 26 percent were male, and only 27.5 percent were married. Over one-fifth had spent time in a nursing home, and nearly half had been in the hospital during the preceding year.

Several points arise from these data. Those receiving care were no more impaired than the entire disabled elderly population as measured by the ADL scale, although those spending $136 or more per month had somewhat higher median ADL scores than the other groups. Family income, however, bore a strong positive relationship to expenditures for home health care. In addition, women and unmarried persons were more likely to hire paid providers. Thus ability to pay and availability of informal caregivers were more important than functional dependency in distinguishing disabled elderly who pay for care from those who receive only unpaid assistance. Finally, it is important to note that the majority of the disabled elderly in the community have nonpaid caregivers, and that only one in twenty receives paid help exclusively.

Marketing: Home health care consumers want convenience,

quality, and low price. Convenience can be facilitated by offering consumers one-stop shopping: a single phone call accesses all aspects of home health care—assessment, counseling, provision of all services and equipment. The agency itself may provide all, some, or none of these, acting as a case coordinator for the patient and subcontracting for services or equipment that it does not offer. Quality is an elusive factor that nearly all care providers claim to possess. Patients are likely to assess quality care from the pleasantness and apparent competence of the nurse or aide and from their perception of the sponsoring hospital's reputation. Price is relative to competitors and other sources of care. Market rates for private-pay consumers are generally from 25 to 75 percent below Medicare rates, and increasing competition is likely to drive them even lower.

A typical hospital-based home health care program gets about three-fourths of its patients from the parent hospital, with the rest coming from the community. However, this proportion varies a great deal, often depending on the marketing efforts of the agency. The hospital discharge planner is usually the referral source for the patient receiving home care immediately after leaving the institution. Just because a home health care agency is affiliated with a hospital does not mean that the hospital's discharge planner will refer any or all potential home care users to that agency; therefore it is wise to establish and maintain relations with discharge planners from all local hospitals.

Of patients seeking care from the community, primary recommenders for home health care agencies are physicians, pharmacists, conservators, community leaders—especially those affiliated with health-related organizations, such as the Red Cross—and clergy. About 70 percent of private home health care arrangements are made by patients' families; only 10 percent are made by professional referral sources. Since the decision-maker in most of these instances is not the patient but the family—most often the daughter or daughter-in-law of the patient—it is the adult children of the frail or disabled elderly at whom marketing efforts should be directed. Other targets should be the well elderly, who may need home care for their friends or themselves at some point; local providers, including pharmacists; legal and financial advisors with elderly clients; and community leaders.

A home health care program should not underestimate the importance of marketing to physicians. A Health Care Financing Administration (HCFA) background paper examining hospital discharges during 1983 and 1984 found that just 3 percent of acute hospital discharges were referred to home care services. More than 5 percent were released to skilled nursing facilities, and about 81 percent were discharged to their homes without home care. Physicians are not always knowledgeable about the availability and value of home health care services and may be unaware that Medicare reimburses for some such services.

Competition: Direct competition for hospital-based home health care programs comes from three sources: (1) other hospital-based agencies, (2) local non-hospital-based firms (proprietary or not-for-profit), and (3) national home care chains. Other hospitals will compete primarily for patients living in the community or just leaving nursing homes, but it is not uncommon for inpatients to be discharged to their homes under the care of a competing home care agency. Since hospital-based programs often have a marketing advantage in terms of perceived quality, other such programs are the toughest competitors when selection is based on care quality.

Of local non-hospital-based firms, proprietary agencies are growing the fastest: between 1979 and 1984, the number of for-profit Medicare-certified home health agencies increased ninefold. Private agencies tend to focus on the non-Medicare market. National chains, such as Upjohn, Quality Care, and Caremark, are growing rapidly; Upjohn has over 300 offices in the United States and abroad. Hospital-based agencies tend to have the most difficulty competing on price with national chains and with low-cost niche players. National chains enjoy substantial economies of scale and sometimes offer proprietary or semiproprietary high-tech home care technology.

Hospital-based programs have advantages over other agencies by dint of their unique role in the referral system. Most consumers think of hospitals when they think of local health care. Moreover, since most home health care patients have recently left a hospital, the discharging institution has a major competitive advantage in promoting its home care program. Hospitals may also have better access to volunteer services that are useful in certain forms of home health care.

Hospitals also have an advantage by dint of size. The recent shifts in the industry showed a marked trend toward survival of the large: most of the agencies that have closed in the last few years have been small. Most of those that have opened or survived have been larger.

The PPS legislation provided incentives for hospitals to establish home health agencies, increased Medicare reimbursement for hospital overhead, and presented an opportunity for hospitals to form joint ventures with agencies. In fact, only hospital-based agencies, gaining 11.6 percent, showed any growth in the 1986–1988 period. In 1983, some 700 hospitals offered home health services. By 1987 the number was over 2000. By 1988, hospitals ran 32 percent of all Medicare-certified agencies, with a typical hospital-based agency conducting 81,000 visits annually.

According to the Health Care Financing Administration, visiting nurses associations (VNAs), which are the primary not-for-profit community-based home care agencies found in most cities, provided more Medicare-reimbursed home health care visits than any other type of agency during 1983. Visiting nurse associations averaged 26 visits per patient, compared with a 33-visit median for proprietary agencies. Proprietary home health agencies also had the highest average total charge *per patient* served ($1675), while hospital-based agencies had the highest average total charge *per visit* ($56) that year. Since 1983, hospital-based and proprietary home care programs have gained market share at the expense of VNAs and other community-based providers.

Timetable: The development of a hospital-based home health care program may take from six to twelve months to reach full operation and Medicare certification. Initial planning and market analysis may require three months, with another three to six months of development activities before services are actually delivered. Medicare licensing usually takes three to nine months. These time frames, with the exception of Medicare certification, will vary widely, depending on how quickly a hospital can act.

A major consideration in funding a home care program is the amount of time spent providing services before reimbursement begins. Receipt of a provider number from Medicare takes a minimum of 60 days, and actual reimbursement from the fiscal intermediary takes at least another month. Since Medicare must observe an operating program before granting a provider number, it is rare for a home care firm to receive reimbursement less than six months after starting to provide services; a year or more is not uncommon. Thus, the sponsoring hospital must be prepared to finance $500,000 to $1,000,000 in receivables to start a home health care program.

Management: Most home health care agencies are separated from hospitals on financial, organizational, and legal bases. This is because the delivery of home care is a different business from providing acute inpatient care. The office itself may be located outside of the hospital, since customer walk-in traffic is not important.

Hospitals may develop or purchase a home health care agency, or joint-venture with an existing organization. Development has the advantages of greater control over the design and higher trust levels among the hospital community, but the process itself is the most time-consuming. This is sometimes the only reasonable decision, since there may be a dearth of available or desirable home care firms to buy or collaborate with.

Purchase of an existing agency may be a feasible option, especially since a hospital is often the primary feeder for the local home care organization and, thus, has substantial bargaining power. This negotiating advantage also holds for purchasing or subcontracting to DME firms. The purchase option obviates the need for the time- and energy-consuming Medicare certification process. However, some hospitals have had difficulty merging their institutional philosophy and culture with those of the acquired agency, which may be a smaller, more entrepreneurial organization. In states with certificate-of-need (CON) laws restricting the number of home health care agencies, however, purchase may be the only option.

Joint venture allows a rapid entrance into the home health care industry at a relatively low cost and low risk. However, this path affords less control and a smaller share of the profits than do the other options. In addition, cultural clash may be a problem with joint ventures. Many hospitals reason that since they will need home care expertise on a relatively permanent basis, it is worth the additional time, capital, and risk to bring that skill inhouse.

Development Concerns: Most hospital-based home health care agencies will want to serve Medicare patients, since reimbursement is adequate and the market is a natural. It is critical that the program be structured so as to maximize the benefits of Medicare reimbursement. Medicare reimburses home care on the lower of costs or charges, which usually means a reasonable cost basis with a cap. If non-Medicare revenues are included within the same organization, overhead will be allocated according to a Medicare formula, which generally is unfavorable to the agency. The best way to work with these restrictions is to erect a tripartite organizational structure, with a Medicare arm, a private-pay arm, and a management arm. Some agencies combine the latter two branches and incorporate the program separately.

The Medicare segment provides only Medicare-reimbursable services. The private-pay segment provides all non-Medicare services and subcontracts any services that the agency does not offer directly, such as certain types of therapy or DME. The management arm provides administrative services to the other two sections for a fee. Although the management section technically breaks even, it is the vehicle through which overhead can be spread over the Medicare arm of the agency.

Home health care firms in many states face regulatory issues in addition to Medicare certification. As of 1985, 34 states had CON requirements for new home health care agencies. An FTC staff report found that home care costs on average were 2 percent higher in areas with CON regulations than in unregulated areas.

In addition to the structuring of the program, the timing of service availability is also important. If the agency intends to offer one-stop shopping, either through its own services or through subcontracting, then this convenience should be available as soon as the organization begins accepting phone calls. Some agencies have unwisely started by offering only limited services, causing frustrated consumers and providers to look elsewhere for care. Once a reputation is blemished in this way, it often is difficult to convince the marketplace to give the agency another chance.

Increasing competition and decreasing reimbursement seem likely in the home care industry's future. Most industry observers predict the introduction of prospective payment and the elimination of the hospital-based add-on during the coming years.

Information Sources: The National Association for Home Care is the primary industry organization for home health care providers. The address is 519 C Street, N.E., Washington, DC 20002; (202) 547-7424. The Division of Ambulatory Care of the American Hospital Association, at 840 North Lake Shore Avenue, Chicago, IL 60611; (312) 280-6461, is another excellent information source. This organization offers several publications and training seminars designed to aid hospitals in establishing home health care programs.

Other sources include two widely read industry newsletters: *Hospital Home Health*, published by American Health Consultants, 67 Peachtree Park Drive, N.E., Atlanta, GA 30309; (404) 351-4523, and *...Home Health Line*, Port Republic, MD 20676; (301) 586-0100.

The Institute for Health and Aging at the University of California at San Francisco has published the research as *Organizational and Community Responses to Medicare Policy: Summary Results*.

Hospice Care

The modern hospice concept originated in Britain. The term *hospice*, meaning "a resting place for travelers," was chosen to represent something between a hospital and a home. Hospices provide supportive and palliative services for the terminally ill, with the notion of caring for the total patient and family needs. Hospice is a method of care, not a location, and, thus, hospice care can be offered in a hospital, nursing home, freestanding hospice facility, or the patient's home.

Hospice services are intended to allow patients to live out their last days as comfortably and fully as possible and to allow families to participate in and deal with the deaths of their loved ones. Physical, mental, and spiritual needs are considered by an interdisciplinary treatment team. The team often is led by a physician and built around the patient, whose needs and desires are paramount.

Hospice services are medical, psychological, and social. Medical services include treatment focused on the continuing control of symptoms, such as pain and nausea. The pharmacologic technology of pain control is essential to hospice care. Emphasis is placed on relieving mental and physical anguish and encouraging the experience of comfortable living until death. Quality, rather than prolongation, of life, is sought. While most care is delivered outside a general hospital inpatient ward, short-term inpatient care is available in case of crises. A small proportion of patients receive all hospice care on an inpatient basis.

Psychological services include counseling to assist the patient in dealing with death. Often this is provided by a designated nurse or social worker who is particularly skilled at communicating with terminal patients. In addition, bereavement counseling is offered to the family. Some of the counseling is interactive in nature, encouraging the patient and family to openly discuss matters related to the impending death.

Social services include homemaker, home health aide care, and help with arranging final affairs. The former most often apply to those dying at home. Final arrangements may include legal services, financial and estate planning, and even funeral arrangements. The family may be involved in each of these to some extent.

The hospice concept is relatively new to the United States. The nation's first hospice was established in 1973; by 1981, a Joint Commission on Accreditation of Hospitals survey reported 440 operational hospice programs, of which 40 percent were based in hospitals, 23 percent in home health agencies, and 20 percent in some combination. Approximately half of the hospital-based programs had been started during the previous year. By 1988, the number of hospice programs had ballooned to nearly 1700, with programs in every state. According to the National Hospice Organization, 29 percent of these are affiliated with or based in hospitals, 19 percent are associated with home health agencies, 46 percent are independent (providing hospice care only), 2 percent are associated with nursing homes, and the remaining programs are coalition sponsored. According to the National Hospice Organization, 70 percent of Americans know the term *hospice*, but most think it is a place instead of a concept.

Value: Hospices are advantageous for the patients and their families desiring that type of treatment. Terminally ill persons with degenerative conditions choose hospice care because they wish to die with dignity and a minimum of pain. Families receive bereavement counseling and support from persons skilled in providing these difficult services.

Hospices are valuable to sponsoring hospitals for several reasons. They serve as excellent public relations vehicles, since hospices are generally perceived as attempts to humanize medical care. Many consumers also associate the hospice concept with progressive health care, an image that most hospitals would like to possess. Hospitals with hospice programs often are able to derive additional Medicare reimbursement beyond that based on standard inpatient treatment, and also to shorten the DRG-reimbursed length of stay.

Hospices are a link in the referral system and not necessarily the last one: about 15 percent of hospice patients die in a hospital, so the sponsoring institution has a good chance of admitting or readmitting a hospice patient shortly before death. Finally, hospice care is reimbursed under a variety of payment mechanisms, generating revenue and (occasionally) some profit. Profitability usually requires economies of scale associated with hospice programs serving well over 100 patients per year.

Cost: The cost of a hospice program depends largely on the program's form. If the hospice is based inside the hospital, the cost will be similar to a standard inpatient unit. Although the actual medical care generally will be less intense, the counseling needs and staff time involvement will be greater. If the hospice is incorporated into a home health care agency, its costs will be similar to other services provided by the agency, although the service may be more intensive. Likewise, a hospice based in a nursing home will have a cost structure similar to that of its parent institution, with minor variations due to care and counseling intensity.

Staffing: The hospice treatment team is multidisciplinary. At the core of the group is the patient. A physician usually heads the team, which also may include a nurse, a social worker, a spiritual counselor, and one or more volunteers. Typically, staff also available include a psychiatrist or psychologist, a clinical pharmacologist, a radiologist, and a physical therapist.

The staffing levels for a hospice depend on the structure of the program. A typical 45-bed freestanding hospice facility would have a physician director, perhaps two or three part-time physicians, six registered nurses, two licensed practical nurses, a social worker, an admissions registrar, and a director of volunteers. A consultant psychiatrist, a pharmacologist, a radiologist, and a physical therapist would also be available. Several dozen—sometimes several hundred—specially trained volunteers would round out the staff.

A home care hospice program may be coordinated with hospitals in the community and include medical and nursing consultation, family counseling, and pain consultation and therapy on a 24-hour basis. Ideally, all staff members are available on call through a paging service; this is critical both for complete service and for inspiring patient and family confidence. A home care hospice program would be staffed primarily by nurses, with a social worker, an administrator, and a medical director (who could be hired part-time under contract). A smaller hospice program could contract with local home care agencies to provide nursing care. Under this model, staff would include an administrator, a physician and a pharmacist (both of them full time or part-time), a medical social worker, and perhaps a medical records librarian.

A hospital-based hospice would have most specialists on hand, but would still need to train staff and volunteers to work with terminal patients and their families. An eight-bed unit typically would have an administrator, a medical director, a nursing director, a social worker, a minister, and staff nurses; few aides would be used in this setting. Inpatient hospices face the challenge of training staff to deal with terminal patients in ways that would be inappropriate for non-terminal inpatients, but essential for hospice patients. A nursing-home-based hospice would have staffing patterns similar to a freestanding facility, with most specialized skills provided on a counsulting basis via relationships with area hospitals and providers.

Revenues: A typical hospice program serving 100 patients per year could generate $250,000 to $350,000 in annual revenues. Payment comes from Medicare and out-of-pocket expenditures, with Medicaid, private insurance, and other sources providing only small amounts of funding.

Legislation in 1982 made hospice care reimbursable under Medicare on a trial basis; the policy was extended permanently in 1985. Medicare reimburses certified hospices for four types of services: routine home care ($63.17 per day), inpatient care ($281 per day), respite care for families ($65.33 per day), and continuous home care for medical emergencies ($368.67 per 24-hour period). The average cost per patient in a certified hospice cannot exceed a cost cap in a given year; the cap currently is just over $8304, and few hospices are having difficulty keeping average costs below this limit. As of January 1989, there is no limit to the days of coverage. No more than 20 percent of all hospice patient days for a given program may be spent in an inpatient unit. A hospice may not discharge a Medicare patient.

Out-of-pocket reimbursement is structured differently from Medicare reimbursement. Services may be billed on a per-visit or per-day basis. Private insurance coverage is similar to Medicare reimbursement, although there usually is a per-patient cap. According to the National Hospice Organization, there are no flat fees—hospices charge on a per diem basis. In some areas Aetna has a $10,000 cap, Blue Cross/Blue Shield has an $8000 cap.

While only a small number of insurance programs cover hospice care, that number is growing rapidly. According to the National Hospice Organization, two-thirds of American workers are covered by hospice benefits. Most large insurance firms now offer the program to their own employees and large corporate customers. Blue Cross and Blue Shield recently produced model hospice benefit guidelines for their affiliates. According to the National Hospice Organization, 66 percent of American workers are covered by hospice benefits. Colorado, Maryland, Michigan, Nevada, New York, and West Virginia require all insurance companies and group health plans to offer hospice benefits, except for self-insured employers.

Medicaid offers hospice benefits in 14 states with payment rates and program methodology the same as for Medicare. Currently, Medicaid has plans to offer hospice benefits in 10 additional states. Some services delivered in the home are funded by Medicaid, as are many nursing home services. However, the elements of care that are unique to the hospice concept generally are not reimbursed by Medicaid.

Market: The market for hospice services consists primarily of terminal cancer patients and their families. About 90 percent of hospice patients suffer from cancer. Because cancer rates are high among the elderly, and because Medicare is the primary funding source for hospice care, the majority of hospice patients are over the age of 65. According to the National Hospice Organization, the average age of the hospice patient is 55. Forty-nine percent of those receiving hospice care are elderly.

Cancer is not the only disease for which hospice care is appropriate. The fastest-growing market segment for hospice services is AIDS (acquired immune deficiency syndrome) patients, most of whom are under age 65, but nearly all of whom are terminal. Advanced multiple sclerosis, severe heart, kidney, or liver ailments, or other terminal conditions may also represent potential patients. A community of 100,000 can be expected to generate about 100 potential hospice patients over the age of 65 each year and a somewhat smaller number of younger persons. Whether these potential patients eventually seek hospice care depends on their awareness of and interest in the service and their ability to pay for it.

Marketing: Given the newness of the hospice concept, relatively few terminally ill patients seek such care on their own. Thus, marketing efforts should be aimed at individuals who are likely to come in contact with dying persons and who would be in positions to suggest hospice care. Physicians are an ideal market. Because cancer is the most prevalent reason for hospice use, oncologists are the most likely to come in contact with potential patients. Discharge planners are also excellent referral sources, as are human service managers, social workers, and clergy. Because hospice care is not well understood by most people, the marketing effort may take time and sensitivity.

Nursing homes, home health agencies, and other hospitals are potential sources of hospice patients. However, they are also competitors in many respects. Although education about hospice and its distinction from traditional terminal acute care may encourage some referrals, representatives of these organizations may perceive—often correctly—that referring a patient to a hospice reduces their own revenues.

Competition: Competition may come from other hospices in the area: with nearly 1500 hospices nationwide, most communities have at least one program available. Although hospital-based programs may have certain marketing advantages over freestanding or other hospices, collaboration should be considered as an alternative to competition. After all, hospice programs are more likely to lose than to earn money, and the other reasons for establishing such a service—goodwill, inpatient referral, better care for some patients—can be achieved by joining efforts with a nonhospital program.

Traditional acute care services are another source of competition for hospice services. Home health agencies, nursing homes, and other hospitals may compete with a hospital-based hospice. In fact, the sponsoring hospital itself may be competition. Educating potential referral sources, patients, and families may overcome competitive barriers to hospice care.

Timetable: The time required to establish a hospice depends in part on the form of the program. An actual freestanding structure will take longer to construct than a modified hospital ward, which itself will require more time to establish than a home-based program. Whatever the form, a significant amount of time is needed in the premarketing phase. Educating the community and raising funds to support the program (if desired) usually takes six months or more. The Medicare certification process also takes several months to complete.

Management: Elements of hospice care are similar to traditional acute care, but the entire process is fundamentally different. While acute care is intended to save the patient's life, hospice care aims to ease the patient's death within the context of the family unit. These differences usually indicate that hospice management is best done by individuals experienced in this special type of care.

For inpatient hospice care, most hospice managers recommend establishing a separate unit where all staff are specialists. Such a ward would be housed in a hospital but would operate under a routine and set of practices especially designed for terminal care. In terms of home hospice care, management requires an individual with home care experience, but that experience alone does not qualify a manager to coordinate a hospice program.

Development Concerns: A needs assessment for a hospice program should include an age breakdown of the local population, an investigation of cancer incidence, and an exploration of other area hospices. Establishing a hospice is likely to be difficult in a typical community of under 100,000 persons that is already served by at least one program.

Most hospital-based hospices will want to apply for Medicare certification. Approximately 55 percent of existing programs are Medicare-certified, largely because Medicare rates have been lower than private-pay rates and because the Medicare program originally was experimental. However, since Medicare rates have increased, and recent legislation has extended the program indefinitely, more hospices are expected to apply for certification. Hospitals may have an advantage in gaining certification because of the range of available personnel and services provided, as well as their familiarity with government qualification procedures.

A key to an effective and efficient hospice is a sound volunteer program. Volunteers are actively used to help the patient and the family. Tasks performed include respite work, chores, transportation, and perhaps assistance with final arrangements. The typical hospice volunteer is female, middle-aged, and active, but persons of all ages and sexes participate. Some large programs have as many as several hundred volunteers. An efficient use of resources allows the recruiting of volunteers to overlap with marketing the hospice to the community.

Establishing an inpatient hospice unit has risks and benefits for a hospital. Aside from the challenges of managing a different type of care within the hospital walls, a Medicare-certified program must be sure to limit its average inpatient day rate to 20 percent of total patient days. Hospital-based hospices sometimes make the error of viewing the program as an outlet for terminal patients who have exceeded the average DRG reimbursement period. Such hospices will have sicker patients with shorter mean survival times than other programs; a number of these patients will spend their entire stay in the inpatient unit. Bedded hospices making this mistake have run up against the 20 percent limit. However, it is possible to exceed the Medicare limit and still increase total Medicare revenues when both acute and hospice care are taken into account. In addition, as hospital census declines, converting acute care beds to terminal beds becomes increasingly practical; this certainly is less expensive than establishing a freestanding hospice, but more so than developing a program that is primarily home-based.

Information Sources: The National Hospice Organization is the primary industry organization for hospice care; the group's address is 1901 North Fort Myer Drive, Suite 307, Arlington, VA 22209; (703) 243-5900. The staff can provide names and phone numbers of hospice managers for various types of programs around the country. The organization can also supply publications useful to health care planners and persons interested in the hospice concept.

Meals on Wheels and Congregate Meals

Title III-C funding subsidizes nutrition programs for Americans aged 60 or older and their spouses of any age. These funds are administered by state and area agencies on aging, which usually contract with local agencies to provide meals for older adults. Other meal programs are funded wholly or in part by grants and charitable donations.

Nutrition programs either deliver meals to older adults' homes or provide meals in a congregate setting. Although a large proportion of these services are provided by community agencies or religious organizations, hospitals increasingly are becoming involved.

Home-delivered meals, often called "meals on wheels," are intended for older persons who are temporarily or permanently disabled or who cannot themselves purchase and prepare adequate meals. Those needing meal service who are capable of traveling to a congregate setting are encouraged to do so, for reasons of both cost and socialization. Some meals-on-wheels programs can accommodate special dietary needs or preferences, such as diabetic, low-salt, or kosher diets. Meals may be hot or cold, and typically are delivered around lunchtime every weekday.

Meals-on-wheels programs rarely earn a surplus and often are subsidized by the sponsoring organization. Reimbursement from an AAA generally averages about $1 per meal. Meal recipients are encouraged to contribute toward food costs, but this is not required. Most programs use volunteer drivers. A typical hospital-based meals-on-wheels program might serve 50 meals per day, and might have 60 volunteers involved in meal delivery. This varies widely, however: St. Luke's Hospital in San Francisco has a $680,000 contract to provide daily meals, which are delivered by Meals on Wheels of San Francisco to 600 older adults.

Congregate meal programs can take any number of forms. Many community-based services provide lunch or dinner within their own facilities or at local senior centers or religious establishments. A hospital may provide Title III-subsidized meals in its cafeteria, or might simply offer older adults a discount on all cafeteria purchases. These can be attractively packaged: one hospital advertises dinners for elders in a relaxed atmosphere, encouraging socialization while promoting nutritious eating. Although congregate meals programs are unlikely to generate profits, they represent a means to make use of kitchen space and personnel that might otherwise be idle, and, thus, may garner some marginal revenue. Meals programs also link to the sponsoring hospital older adults who may need acute care services in the future.

Information Sources: For more information, contact the National Association of Meals Programs, 204 E Street, N.W., Washington, DC 20002; (202) 547-6157.

St. Mary's Hospital and Medical Center in San Francisco runs a successful congregate meals program for older adults, serving lunch and dinner in the hospital cafeteria seven days a week. For more information about the Gold Card Dining Club, contact the program director at 450 Stanyan Street, San Francisco, CA 94117; (415) 750-5942 or (415) 750-5880.

Medicare Health Maintenance Organizations

Since February of 1985, health maintenance organizations and other competitive medical plans (CMPs) have been authorized to enroll Medicare beneficiaries. This has led to dramatic growth in the number and size of so-called Medicare HMOs, which, due to a law requiring that no more than 50 percent of a sponsoring organization's total membership may be over 65, must be affiliated with HMOs for younger persons.

As of 1988, just over 3 percent of the Medicare population (1.05 million of the over 30 million Medicare beneficiaries) was enrolled in HMOs authorized since 1985. Another 1.7 million beneficiaries were enrolled in HMOs in existence before 1985. The pre-1985 HMOs are reimbursed under a system that the federal government plans to phase out.

During the start-up years for Medicare HMOs, the HCFA was bullish on their enrollment growth. However, in January 1988, Inter-Study, a not-for-profit research and consulting firm, predicted "substantial slowdown in growth" for Medicare HMOs. Plans serving the elderly population report dissatisfaction with the government's reimbursement rates. In addition, some have systems insufficient to control the elderly's utilization of health care services.

In 1988, 29 HMOs discontinued their contracts with Medicare. If reimbursement rates do not improve, more HMOs may drop out of the program in 1989. A recent survey by the Group Health Association of America, a Washington-based association representing HMOs, found 30 percent of 74 HMOs surveyed will not renew their contracts in 1989.

Older adults enjoy several benefits from enrolling in a Medicare HMO. Benefits per dollar spent tend to be greater, and the paperwork that most elderly persons find confusing is reduced. Health maintenance organizations typically offer better care coordination than traditional health plans and, therefore, are good for persons with complicated health conditions. Surveys from the plans that participated in the HCFA's demonstrations conducted in 1980 found that, on average, over 90 percent of participants were satisfied with care quality—a figure that compared favorably to the proportion in the same locations who received care under the traditional payment system. Thus despite the requirement that enrollees choose a physician who participates in the plan, older adults seem enthusiastic about HMOs.

The majority of Medicare HMOs have been started by existing HMOs or insurance companies. However, many hospitals have established HMOs or joint-ventured with existing health plans in efforts to increase their elder market share. Virtually none of these could be described as successful in filling hospital beds. This should not be surprising, since HMOs achieve their cost savings largely by keeping enrollees out of hospitals. However, some hospital-sponsored plans have found HMOs good vehicles to increase physician utilization.

Currently, only 29 percent of Medicare HMOs are profitable, according to a recent survey by InterStudy. The remaining plans reported they were breaking even (20 percent), operating under "somewhat unfavorable" financial conditions (22 percent), or operating under "very unfavorable" conditions (29 percent) (see Figure 3-1).

InterStudy reported Medicare HMOs' perception of their financial risk or success was significantly related to two variables: (1) control of beneficiaries, and (2) hospital utilization and the per-

FIGURE 3-1 _____

Reported Financial Experience of Medicare HMOs

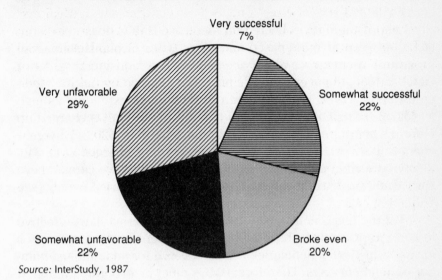

Source: InterStudy, 1987

ceived adequacy of the reimbursement rate. The government reimburses HMOs 95 percent of the adjusted average per capita cost (AAPCC), a formula which takes into account the sex, age, institutional status, welfare status, and geographic location of enrollees.

Some hospital-sponsored Medicare HMOs apparently have suffered from _adverse selection_ of beneficiaries; that is, enrollees have been less healthy than average for the local area. This has resulted in higher utilization and costs than anticipated for some plans. Because the HCFA does not consider the health status of enrollees in the Medicare plans, adverse selection can engender huge losses for an HMO, a fact to which a number of hospital-sponsored plans can attest. An additional issue is the variability of the AAPCC by geographic area, on which payments to HMOs are based. In 1989, the monthly rates per beneficiary for combined hospital and physician services will vary from a high of $420.90 to a low of $118.53 (excluding plans in Guam, the Virgin Islands, and Puerto Rico). The national monthly per capita rate, from which the AAPCC is computed, is $258.60 for 1989. Plans that have lost money have complained that their area payment rates are too low. In addition, some evidence suggests that the AAPCC is a poor surrogate for actual care costs in a given area.

Much of the data collected on Medicare HMOs does not distinguish between hospital-based and other types of plans. Among all programs, premiums and service ranges vary considerably. As of October 1988, the average basic premium charged by the 155 Medicare HMOs was $30.44 per month, with a range extending as high as $64.52. The HCFA reported 10 percent of the HMOs charged no monthly premium, 17 percent charged less than $20, 46 percent charged between $21 and $40, and 46 percent charged over $40. Most plans offered extended hospital days, preventive care and eye care as part of their coverage, but other benefits varied widely (see Table 3-3).

With the enactment of the catastrophic coverage law, effective in 1989, HMOs must change some of the benefits they offer. For example, in 1989 beneficiaries will be covered for an unlimited number of inpatient days. Therefore, HMOs must incorporate unlimited hospital days into their benefit package rather than offering this as an additional service.

Marketing a plan can be the key to its success, not merely to enroll a minimum number of people but also to enroll a population

TABLE 3-3
HMO Services Offered beyond Traditional Medicare Benefits, 1983

Benefit	Plans offering benefit (%)
Unlimited hospital days	94
Extended SNF days	24
Waive hospital and SNF coinsurance	33
Routine physical	87
Immunization	84
Health education	65
Outpatient drugs	28
Eye exam	71
Ear care	62
Dental	15
Outpatient mental health	55

Source: Health Care Financing Administration, Office of Prepared Healthcare, 1984

of older persons that is no sicker than average for its local area. Thus, any promotion to groups with heavy care needs—such as residents of convalescent homes—should be counterbalanced with marketing to healthier than average persons, as might be found at senior recreation clubs. All promotional and informational materials, including brochures and application forms, must be submitted to HCFA for approval at least 45 days before release.

One advantage to a hospital for establishing a Medicare HMO is that it prepares the institution for the day when capitation may be the dominant form of reimbursement for eldercare. Although the experience will differ from coordinating a broad range of care, a Medicare HMO would nonetheless give a hospital practice in working closely with its medical staff in a capitated setting. If and when the eldercare financing system moves toward capitation, such expertise could be very valuable.

Information Sources: Perhaps the best source of information about HMOs is InterStudy, a not-for-profit research and consulting organization located in Minnesota. Each year, InterStudy publishes a data book on Medicare and HMOs. A 1985 publication, *The Future of Medicare and HMOs,* provides a concise analysis of the state of the field as well as recommendations for providers and policymakers. Another excellent resource is InterStudy's 1987 publication, *Risky Business: An examination of TEFRA Risk HMOs and Their Contracting Experience,* which examines the financial experience of 41 Medicare HMOs. InterStudy's address is P.O. Box 458, Excelsior, MN 55331; (612) 474-1176.

Another source of information is the Health Care Financing Administration's Office of Prepaid Healthcare at 330 Independence Avenue, S.W., Room 4360, Washington, DC 20201; (202) 245-0815.

Mental Health Programs

The elderly are at high risk for several mental health problems, most notably depression and organic brain syndromes (the senile dementias). Much evidence indicates that mental disorders are more likely to be undiagnosed in older adults than in other age groups. As many as one-fourth of the elderly population experiences significant mental health problems. Persons over age 65 account for approximately 30 percent of all residents of public mental hospitals, and the majority of these involve conditions onsetting in old age. As many as one-fourth of the elderly population experience significant mental health problems.

The last few decades have seen a conscious government effort to deinstitutionalize mental hospital patients, and although many of the elderly who once were hospitalized have been released, approximately half of those deinstitutionalized from public hospitals were subsequently admitted to nursing homes. For the most part, the funding for deinstitutionalized patients has not followed them into the community or the nursing home.

An estimated 50 to 60 percent of all nursing home residents have either a primary or secondary diagnosis of mental illness. However, the prevalence of mental illness among nursing home residents may be rising because persons entering nursing homes tend to be sicker now as compared to the past. A recent study identified a mental disorder in 94 percent of nursing home residents.

Hospitals can provide a number of mental health services to older adults. Diagnostic services address the high rate of undiagnosed mental illness in the elderly, including dementia, depression, and alcohol and drug abuse. Diagnostic services include health screening and health assessment programs. Preventive services include mental, social, and perceptual stimulation, as well as education; these can be incorporated into many personal and long-term eldercare services. Crisis services make mental health professionals available by phone or in emergency rooms to identify and respond to acute mental health crises. Protective services are essential for older adults who may not be responsible for their actions, and include both hands-on care or observation and installation of safety features in homes.

Mental health services can be delivered in a variety of settings. Acute inpatient services, which are not ideal for the chronic mental problems of many older adults, are nonetheless appropriate in some cases. Psychiatric consultations combined with acute care may improve the clinical outcome of the elderly patient. Recent studies show that mental health interventions can both significantly reduce the length of stay and improve the clinical outcome of hospitalized elderly cardiac and surgery patients. Services might be delivered within a general hospital psychiatric unit or in a special psychiatric hospital. Either of these sites can also offer outpatient services, as might freestanding short-stay community psychiatric centers; the largest growth in mental health service utilization has been in community-based and outpatient psychiatric services. Adult day care and respite care programs usually serve a large proportion of older adults.

A special type of mental health program treats only Alzheimer's disease, either in a nursing home or through a day care program. Because the prevalence of Alzheimer's disease and other severe dementias rises with age, the number of cases will multiply as seniors live longer. The Office of Technology Assessment estimates that the number of cases will increase 58 percent by 2020, to 3.3 million from 1.4 million in 1980.

The OTA estimates there are as many as 200 Alzheimer nursing homes in the nation, designed to enable patients to function at their highest possible levels. Estimates vary because of a lack of consensus on the definition of special care units. Despite the proliferation of special care units, only a small percentage of elderly with dementia are treated in these units. The OTA reports that 1 to 2 percent of nursing home residents with severe dementia are in special care units. However, the number of residents suffering from dementia may be as high as 60 percent, according to some studies.

These units generally cost $5 to $15 more per day than other nursing home care. Staffing levels tend to be 15 to 20 percent larger than average. These programs can be quite profitable, particularly if the unit treats a high ratio of private-pay patients. Proprietary chains, including Beverly Enterprises, Manor Care, National Medical Enterprises' Hillhaven Corporation, and ARA Services are rushing into the field. In 1987, Hillhaven opened the first nursing home for Alzheimer's patients only.

Individuals with dementia are more likely to spend down to Medicaid eligibility because they have lengthy nursing home stays, according to the OTA. Neither the Medicaid nor Medicare programs have special entitlements for individuals with dementia.

Information Sources: The Northwestern Memorial Hospital Institute of Psychiatry, at 259 East Erie Street, Chicago, IL 60611, has both inpatient and outpatient mental health services for older adults. For more information about inpatient services contact the program director at (312) 908-7460; for outpatient services, call (312) 908-7460.

An interesting program that provides consultation and therapy for older adults is sponsored by Good Samaritan Hospital in Puyallup, Washington. Contact Good Samaritan Outreach Services at 407 14th Avenue, S.E., Puyallup, WA 98372; (206) 848-5571.

The Alzheimer's and Related Disorders Association of Chicago has a useful publication, *Selecting a Nursing Home with a Dedicated Dementia Care Unit*, for a nominal charge.

Personal Emergency Response Systems

Many frail elderly patients, particularly those who live alone, are kept in the hospital or nursing home longer than treatment and recovery would require because of the risk involved with sending them home. Many of these individuals do not need medical or even supportive care, but nonetheless are quite vulnerable should an emergency occur. Some patients who do return home are plagued by anxiety about relapses or accidents. Personal emergency response systems (PERS) address these needs. The American Hospital Association reports that close to two-thirds of community hospitals surveyed have some form of PERS program.

Personal emergency response systems provide at-risk elderly persons effective and convenient means to summon help when an emergency occurs. Usually the person wears or carries a *transmitter unit* so that even in the event of a crippling fall or stroke, the patient is capable of activating an alarm. Pushing a button on the transmitter activates the unit on the telephone, which seizes the phone line and dials the 24-hour response center. The transmitter unit identifies the individual having an emergency. Typically, the hospital staff member checks the subscriber's file, which contains the person's name, address, medication information, physician, and names and numbers of emergency responders—designated relatives or friends who live nearby and have a key to the subscriber's residence.

Once the hospital staff is notified of a problem, either through inactivity or a help signal, a staff member calls the residence to check if the signal was transmitted accidentally. This more often than not is the case. If there is no response at the subscriber's home, the first emergency responder is called. The responder calls the hospital immediately upon arriving at the subscriber's home to summon a rescue vehicle if necessary. Many programs call all clients on a monthly basis to test the system and confirm the information on file.

An innovative variation on the system involves direct voice communication. An *enhanced speakerphone* with a 50-foot range is built into the central unit and attached to the subscriber's phone, allowing direct communication with the sponsoring organization. If an emergency occurs outside of voice range, the emergency responder is called to check on the subscriber. Voice communication systems often encourage nonemergency social calls to address the needs of the socially isolated older person.

Many PERS services also have a backup system in the form of an *inactivity timer.* This device must be activated at regular intervals, perhaps one or more times each day, or after completion of a task, such as opening the refrigerator or using the bathroom. If the unit is untouched at the designated time, a message will alert the resident that it is preparing to phone the hospital. This provides the forgetful subscriber a chance to deactivate the device, but, if appropriate, the system will summon aid for the incapacitated patient.

There are several thousand personal emergency response programs nationwide, most of them based in hospitals. Lifeline, the oldest and largest of the organizations selling PERS, has 2200 client hospitals and has sold over 200,000 transmitter units. Systems have evolved over the past decade, with three forms emerging.

1. A *local system* is usually hospital-based. Subscribers rent or lease the transmitter units from the hospital. The hospital houses the communications center, usually located in the emergency room area.

2. A *national system* is usually coordinated by the firm manufacturing the system components. Subscribers rent or

lease the transmitter units from the hospital; emergency messages are sent to a national response center, which then contacts the local hospital and first responders.

3. An *individual system* is managed by the system designer. The transmitter units are sold directly to individuals, who can designate the parties to be alerted in case of emergency.

These options are listed in decreasing order of hospital involvement. In the local system, a hospital is responsible for coordinating the program, marketing the service, notifying first responders, and answering the call. In a national structure, the hospital markets the service and responds to the alert. When the units are sold directly to individual users, the hospital is not part of a system but merely responds to the electronically generated message—if it is a designated recipient. The local system is by far the most prevalent, but the other types of programs are growing in share.

Value: The value of a PERS to a frail individual is immense. It allows a patient to return home from a hospital or nursing home earlier than would otherwise be safe or desirable, and it allows some individuals to stay out of a nursing facility entirely. Personal emergency response systems have saved countless lives by summoning help quickly. Even more commonly, such programs have eased the anxiety of many at-risk older persons and their families worried about vulnerability to accident or sudden illness. In addition, voice communication systems provide a social connection for subscribers.

The value of a PERS program to a hospital also is high. The most visible benefit is the program's public relations value. Sponsoring a PERS program usually is perceived as an indication of institutional commitment to serving the elderly beyond the hospital walls. The system also furthers a hospital's mission to provide care to the community members who need assistance most: the frail elderly. Emergency medical response systems are excellent "high-tech, high-touch" marketing mechanisms, increasing the likelihood that subscribers will use the sponsoring hospital when institutionalization is required.

Emergency medical response programs also can be financially rewarding for a hospital. While a majority of hospital-based systems do not turn a profit, many do, depending on the local marketplace and the prices charged. Regardless of profitability, the indirect savings can be substantial. A strong PERS program allows patients to be discharged earlier than would otherwise be possible, generating significant savings under DRG-based reimbursement. Increased utilization due to the emergency medical connection is another indirect financial benefit, although this typically is fairly small.

Cost: The cost to a hospital of establishing a personal emergency response system is relatively modest, given the benefits. A locally based, 25-unit Lifeline system, for instance, can be established for about $20,000. If purchased with 20 or more transmitter units, the hospital-based communications center costs about $5000, and each unit costs from $500 to $700, depending on features. Most hospitals begin their programs with 20 to 25 units ($10,000 to $17,500) and increase their inventories by about 20 units per year. Lifeline reports that the median hospital-based program has between 100 and 125 units.

A centrally operated direct voice communications system, such as Communicalls, saves the costs of the communications center, since the vendor monitors all calls via a WATS (wide area telephone service) line. Transmitter unit costs average about $600, and the monthly monitoring fee is $20 to $25. Such a system involves marketing and billing costs, but no extra staffing to operate the system itself.

Even for a hospital-based PERS program, staffing costs are likely to be minimal, especially since much of the work can be performed by volunteers. A sponsoring hospital will need to install a designated telephone for the communications center and usually will install an additional reserved outgoing line as well; these costs also tend to be small. Marketing costs for brochures and advertising may add up to a few thousand dollars at the outside. In addition, most personal emergency response system vendors are eager to assist with public relations and marketing efforts.

Staffing: The nature of personal emergency response systems requires a minimal level of staffing. A PERS program generally is operated out of a hospital emergency room. The program is unlikely to require staff time other than workers specifically assigned to the program. A program with 100 subscribers typically would answer

40 to 50 emergency calls per year, or an average of one per week. Thus, the establishment of an emergency response system does not require enlarging the hospital emergency room staff. If a hospital participates in a nationally based system, even less staff time is involved.

A personal emergency response program requires a designated coordinator, but that person may be assigned half-time or less. Most hospital-based programs use a social worker, nurse, emergency room clerk, director of volunteers, or director of communication services to coordinate the system. The bulk of other workers are volunteers, who may help by checking and updating subscriber files, marketing the program through community organizations, and fund-raising (if necessary). The system vendor often helps to train staff.

Revenues: The direct revenues for a PERS program come from rental or lease fees for the transmitter units. Hospitals typically charge between $25 and $35 per unit. If the market will bear fees in the upper half of those ranges, it is possible for the hospital to earn a profit on the program. A 25-unit program priced at $20 per month would gross $6000 per year, or $9000 annually for a $30-per-month voice communication system, assuming all units were rented at all times. This is quite possible; many smaller hospital-based programs have waitlists for transmitter units, although others aim for less than full utilization so as to have units available at all times for those in need.

Some PERS programs receive support from grants or foundations. Others raise funds from individuals and businesses in the community. The popularity and visibility of PERS programs makes them excellent candidates for fund-raising from a variety of sources. For example, local businesses pay to have their name on one or more of the transmitter units; at $500 to $700 per unit, it is a relatively inexpensive yet highly visible public relations gesture.

Emergency care services generated by PERS programs usually are reimbursable under Medicare, Medicaid, or private third-party insurance. Some of the services may be paid for out of pocket. The PERS services themselves are rarely reimbursed by public or private third-party sources, although a small number of insurers and HMOs pay for patients at risk for accidents. Medicaid is currently operating demonstration projects in 17 states and eventually may reimburse for personal emergency response services.

Market: The market for personal emergency response systems consists of frail or disabled persons, primarily those living alone. On average, about 3 percent of elderly persons in a community, and 0.6 percent of those under age 65, have health conditions that make them potential PERS users. Thus, a hospital with a service area population of 50,000 would typically have a market of 150 to 200 elderly persons and several hundred more below age 65. Market penetration of 5 percent would support a program with 20 to 25 transmitter units. Users typically are female with an average age in the late seventies.

Marketing: A critical marketing target is the hospital discharge planner. Most potential PERS users can be identified well before discharge; many can even be designated upon admission. For instance, an elderly woman living alone with a history of falling would appear to be at risk for the type of emergency that PERS are designed to address. Discharge planners at the sponsoring and surrounding hospitals should be aware of the system and its capabilities.

Often hospital-based programs advertise in local newspapers or church or community newsletters. Many PERS vendors supply sample advertising copy and some offer cooperative advertising programs in which the cost of the ad is split between the hospital and the manufacturer. Volunteers and staff members often make presentations about the program for senior organizations, religious institutions, clubs, or even provider groups. In addition, much marketing for personal emergency response systems is done by word of mouth.

Competition: Other hospitals or community-based programs may compete for PERS customers. Some home health agencies, area agencies on aging, and meals-on-wheels programs may sponsor PERS program. However, most other hospitals will not encroach directly on a program's catchment area, given that customers are likely to prefer establishing a PERS relationship with the closest institution.

There is reason to believe that the presence of other nearby PERS is beneficial for all concerned. Hospitals with waitlists for transmitter units often refer interested consumers to nearby programs that are not full. Moreover, the first PERS program in an area will introduce the concept to the community, reducing the marketing necessary for subsequent programs. Thus, the presence of locally based competition is not necessarily a cause for concern in the PERS field.

Potentially, manufacturers that sell units directly to consumers or through nonhospital distribution centers, such as home security system retailers, could represent a competitive threat to a hospital-based personal emergency response system. Presently, few such sales have been made. However, experts predict that direct marketing to consumers will increase in the future, although hospital-based systems are expected to dominate the PERS field for the foreseeable future.

Timetable: Emergency medical response systems require relatively little time to establish. Researching the vendors, adding one or two designated phone lines, installing the emergency medical response center, and participating in vendor training sessions can all be completed in about one month. Premarketing can start before the system is fully installed.

Once the program begins, the hospital can expect unit rentals and system usage to start relatively quickly. Once subscribers enter the system, within 18 months approximately 30 percent will use the PERS at least once, and some will use it many times. Vendor-monitored systems may be started more quickly, although the hospital will typically see only one or two additional emergency calls per month due to the introduction of the PERS program.

Management: The key management issue for personal emergency response services is whether to manage the system within the hospital or to enlist in a centrally based, national PERS program. The former gives the hospital more control; the latter requires less capital outlay and staff time. A national program leases transmitter units to hospitals, which then market the program to the local community. Usually the hospital is responsible for billing subscribers.

National programs enjoy economies of scale, allowing cost savings to be passed on to subscribers. However, emergency alert involves an additional step in such programs. A hospital-based system is more appealing to most consumers, who are more comfortable with the notion of their cries for help being heard by a nearby, familiar hospital rather than by an office in another part of the country. Most hospitals in the past have chosen to operate personal emergency response systems themselves, although this is changing.

Development Concerns: A needs assessment and competitor analysis should precede the purchase or lease of a PERS program. Although competition does not preclude the establishment of a personal emergency response program, it is important to know the extent and pricing of nearby systems. Most hospital-based PERS programs will want to start with 20 to 30 transmitter units. Additional units can be purchased as need becomes evident.

Vendor selection is important in establishing a program. Like any endeavor involving a technology-based product, it is crucial that the manufacturer of a PERS system should have service personnel in the local area who can respond to reported problems quickly. Elderly persons who have come to rely on their PERS often become quite anxious when the system breaks down. Similarly, the financial stability of the vendor should be investigated to protect the hospital and subscribers from losing service in the future.

Information Sources: Lifeline, a not-for-profit organization based in the Boston area, is the nation's oldest and largest manufacturer of personal emergency response systems. Contact Lifeline at 1 Arsenal Marketplace, Watertown, MA 02172; (800) 451-0525.

A major vendor of centrally monitored direct voice communication systems is Health Care Technology Corporation, which produces Communicalls. The address and phone number are 295 Treadwell Street, Hamden, CT 06514; (800) 841-3800.

For a nonvendor's view of personal emergency response systems, contact ECRI in Plymouth Meeting, PA; (215) 825-6000. ECRI, a not-for-profit health care equipment-testing organization, recently completed a major background paper on PERS products.

Phone Reassurance and Friendly Visitor Services

Other ways that hospitals can help older adults live independently include phone reassurance and friendly visitor services. In the former, hospital volunteers make regular phone calls to frail elders who are living alone. Those who are recently retired or widowed or who are recovering from an illness may find this service particularly helpful. Calls may be made on an infrequent basis for social purposes or may be made at a specified time each day to check on a person's condition.

A friendly visitor program serves similar purposes. Volunteers stop by an older adult's home one or more times a week to chat and make sure that the client is well. The visitor also may provide some type of assistance, but that is not the focus of the service.

Most hospitals provide phone reassurance and friendly visitor services free of charge through their volunteer programs. The services enable some older adults to live independently who otherwise might be apprehensive about doing so. Both programs generate positive publicity for the sponsoring hospital at very little cost, and serve to connect to the hospital elders who may need medical care at some point.

Information Sources: Walter O. Boswell Memorial Hospital in Sun City, Arizona, offers both phone reassurance and friendly visitor services through its volunteer program. More information is available from the Volunteer Department at P.O. Box 1690, 10401 Thunderbird Boulevard, Sun City, AZ 85372; (602) 876-5387.

Alta Bates/Herrick Hospital and Health Center has a free phone reassurance program called Tele-Care. Their address and phone number are 2001 Dwight Way, Berkeley, CA 94704; (415) 540-4487.

Rehabilitation

Due to demographic and financial changes, rehabilitation services for the elderly are beginning to receive more attention from the health care industry. Americans are starting to realize that, for example, a 65-year-old stroke victim may have 20 to 30 more years of life ahead. Therefore, rehabilitation, once thought to be important primarily for the young, is increasingly being perceived as worthwhile for older adults.

Another impetus for geriatric rehabilitation involves federal reimbursement mechanisms. When the Health Care Financing Administration introduced the prospective pricing system based on diagnosis-related groups for Medicare in 1983, it also established a special system for patients requiring rehabilitation. Hospitals initiating a *distinct part Medicare rehabilitation unit* are allowed additional reimbursement for eligible inpatients beyond the DRG-based limit (i.e., they are considered DRG-exempt for the services delivered on the separate unit). As PPS has been phased in, incentives for hospitals to establish Medicare rehabilitation programs have grown. To date, 591 institutions have developed distinct part units, and more are considering doing so. In addition to these, the nation has 99 dedicated rehabilitation hospitals.

Rehabilitation services generally focus on speech, physical, and occupational therapy. Efforts aimed at restoration of function generally do not begin until the precipitating acute episode—if any— has subsided, and, therefore, skilled nursing care plays a somewhat smaller role, and special therapies a larger role, in rehabilitation compared with most other acute inpatient services.

Older adults can undergo medical rehabilitation in any of a number of sites. Besides designated inpatient units, some services are delivered in other locations within the hospital, at freestanding rehabilitation hospitals, or within a nursing home. In addition, outpatient rehabilitation can be conducted through a day rehabilitation hospital program or through a comprehensive outpatient rehabilitation facility (CORF). Finally, some services are delivered in the home. The various settings have more in common in terms of clinical treatment than management considerations. This section will focus on managing distinct part inpatient Medicare units, although it should be kept in mind that most hospitals with such units also have related outpatient programs.

Value: Rehabilitation services benefit the elderly by allowing victims of crippling conditions to regain some portion of their lost function. This may involve teaching an older person to cope better with an increasingly painful chronic problem, such as rheumatoid arthritis, or training an acutely disabled individual, such as a stroke victim, to relearn speech and motor skills. Whatever the ailment being treated, rehabilitation is intended to restore as much function as possible to the older patient so that he or she can live more years in the best attainable health.

A rehabilitation program benefits a hospital in several respects. First, it provides revenue-generating but non-DRG use for some number of beds, beds that might otherwise be empty. Second, it helps position the hospital as having special expertise in eldercare.

Finally, a DRG-exempt inpatient rehabilitation unit dovetails nicely with other rehabilitation efforts both inside and outside the hospital, and can be directed at both older and younger patients.

The value of a distinct part Medicare unit depends somewhat on each hospital's unique situation. Those with caseloads that are primarily non-Medicare probably will not need a designated unit, since private insurance reimburses for rehabilitation for most younger persons. Hospitals with average lengths of Medicare stay that exceed regional averages will gain more than others from establishing a special section, because they will save on unreimbursed general inpatient costs. Institutions that see a large number of trauma patients are more likely to have a sizable population of patients who could potentially benefit from rehabilitation services, although older adults are less likely than younger persons to be trauma victims.

Cost: Capital expenditure is not a major issue for DRG-exempt rehabilitation units in hospitals that already have general rehabilitation services. Significant renovations probably will not be necessary in order to establish a special section. Primary expenses will involve purchase of some special equipment, but physical changes probably will be minor.

On average, operating costs for an inpatient Medicare rehabilitation unit are roughly equivalent to those for a standard inpatient section that serves primarily older persons, but this varies with the caseload. Stroke victims tend to be less costly to treat than many other patients. Units caring for trauma or major orthopedic conditions may have relatively high costs. Labor expenses are the primary determinants of cost, and they depend largely on the case mix. Because most DRG-exempt sections are on floors housing other medical-surgical units, many overhead expenditures will be shared.

Staffing: Staffing ratios (the number of staff members divided by the number of patients present) tend, on average, to be similar for designated Medicare units and general medical units, but again the caseload causes this to vary. One nurse might oversee five to ten stroke victims, while that same nurse could care for just two or three spinal cord patients, who generally have high care needs.

Rehabilitation units, relative to general medical units, utilize a larger number of rehabilitation nurses and therapists. The latter generally are paid somewhat less than the average registered nurse. One hospital's 21-bed rehabilitation unit has eight professional nurses and another eight nonprofessional nursing staff members.

Medicare rehabilitation units must be overseen by a medical director who must have an M.D. and must devote at least 20 hours per week to the unit. A certified rehabilitation nurse often serves as administrator. Ideally, a physiatrist (a physician specializing in rehabilitative medicine) will be on staff or available for consultation. Physical therapists probably play the largest role in rehabilitation, with speech, occupational, and recreational therapists also quite involved. One or more social workers will work with the program to facilitate reentry into the family and community. Many programs include a part- or full-time audiologist as well.

Currently, many rehabilitation staff members are young, often between 25 and 35 years old. Training is necessary for them to understand the difficulties that older adults often suffer in recovering from a major illness. Staff also must be prepared to deal with the older person who is unwilling to put effort into recovering function, preferring to live (or die) with the disability. Maintaining staff morale is one of the most challenging aspects of managing a Medicare rehabilitation unit. Some hospitals address the issue through in-service training and by rotating staff out of the section every six months.

Revenues: Virtually all revenues for a designated geriatric rehabilitation unit will be associated with the Medicare program; most will come directly from Medicare, with the copayments and deductibles paid out-of-pocket and by Medicaid. Reimbursement is determined by a cost-based formula, rather than by a prospective pricing system. Rehabilitation units tend to support themselves, and some are profitable.

In most areas, all potential rehabilitation patients must be prescreened by a peer review organization (PRO). Experience will quickly tell which types of patients are likely to be approved and which may be denied by the local PRO. For example, stroke patients are commonly recommended for rehabilitation, while those suffering from orthopedic impairments such as hip fractures are routinely denied certification in many localities but sometimes approved in others. Peer review organizations differ widely in their familiarity with rehabilitation, and this experience affects denial rates. Once a patient is approved by a PRO, Medicare will reimburse for treatment.

Market: The population most likely to use inpatient rehabilitation services are inpatients themselves. Rehabilitation units typically receive most—if not all—of their patients from acute care units. Patients may enter the rehabilitation section once their acute condition stabilizes.

In many hospitals, rehabilitation services are performed in a number of different departments. For example, the DRG-exempt rehabilitation unit at Mount Sinai Hospital in Miami Beach, Florida, does not perform cardiovascular rehabilitation because it is handled by the cardiology department.

Stroke tends to be the most common diagnosis on most Medicare rehabilitation units. Orthopedic conditions, Parkinson's disease, multiple sclerosis, and severe rheumatoid arthritis also cause many patients to seek rehabilitation. A typical patient will remain on a rehabilitation unit for between two and six weeks, and then receive outpatient treatment for another six months. By that point, most patients will have achieved perhaps 80 percent of their potential gains.

Marketing: A baseline for demand for rehabilitation services can be projected from local hospital discharge data, which usually is available from municipal or state agencies, or from local or regional health care data consortia. The number of strokes, amputations, joint replacements, and injuries among persons over age 65 should be used to project potential demand for rehabilitation services. For example, out of every 100 stroke victims, between 55 and 85 might be candidates for inpatient rehabilitation. Another demand assessment technique is based on area population. For example, South Dakota estimates the need for 15 rehabilitation beds per every 100,000 residents. Estimates for other states and regions are only now being generated by health systems agencies around the country. It is important to realize that demand projections vary markedly from community to community, depending largely on the familiarity with rehabilitation services of local residents and physicians, and, to a lesser degree, to restrictive state bed regulations.

Target market segments include potential patients and their families, physicians, nurses, social workers, and discharge planners. Although patients and physicians are frequently targeted by hospital promotional campaigns, nurses, social workers, and discharge planners working with patients with rehabilitation potential on medical-surgical units often are overlooked. Marketing efforts should include these professionals, perhaps through personal contact and educational forums. These individuals should be kept informed of the progress of each referred patient because referrals to acute inpatient rehabilitation units often follow patterns. Successful rehabilitation experiences communicated back to the referral sources may result in six to twelve additional referrals each year per source.

Many Medicare rehabilitation programs do not actively promote their services because demand for their beds exceeds supply. Some states restrict the number of rehabilitation beds that can be operated, ensuring that all available programs will be full. While, on average, the nation is underbedded for Medicare rehabilitation services, the supply-demand equation varies greatly by state and by area.

Competition: Competition for inpatient rehabilitation units may come from similar units at other hospitals, or from nursing homes, CORFs, freestanding outpatient rehabilitation facilities, or home health care agencies. In areas where demand for services exceeds supply, competition does not threaten individual rehabilitation programs. In other communities, competitive pressures can be severe.

Nursing homes may provide the most serious form of competition. Although patients and their families generally prefer treatment in a hospital rather than a nursing home, Medicare reimbursement policies often will dictate that care be delivered in the latter. Medicare usually will reimburse for rehabilitation delivered in a skilled nursing facility so long as improvement can be demonstrated. Some patients who are not certified for hospital inpatient rehabilitation treatment will qualify for reimbursement in a skilled nursing facility.

Timetable: The amount of time required to establish a DRG-exempt inpatient rehabilitation unit depends in part on the nature of the facility that will house the section. If it already is fitted for rehabilitation, little or no renovation will be necessary. If not, equipment purchase and structural refitting may take a few months.

The most significant timing issue involves Medicare regulations. The DRG exclusions for inpatient rehabilitation units can only become effective at the start of a hospital's fiscal year. For hospitals converting standard acute beds to rehabilitation, DRG exclusion cannot take effect until at least 75 percent of the converted beds have been used for ten designated diagnoses over the previous 12 months. This restriction does not apply to new beds.

A feature common to all geriatric rehabilitation units is the Medicare review process. This is conducted by a state regulatory agency, which should be notified 60 days before the unit is to be opened as a distinct-part operation, that is, 60 days prior to the start of a hospital's fiscal year. However, the review can be performed in as little time as a week or so if necessary. Survey results typically are received by the hospital about two weeks later. Regulations differ somewhat for new and converted facilities; the state review agency is the best source of information about this and other issues of licensing and government reimbursement.

Management: Because inpatient rehabilitation is relatively similar to many other inpatient services, the challenges faced by administrative management of a distinct part unit do not differ greatly from those involved with managing other units. Clinical management is different, however, since much of the activity on a rehabilitation unit involves helping patients perform tasks for themselves rather than doing things for them. A rehabilitation section typically is overseen by a medical director and a rehabilitation administrator, who often is a certified rehabilitation nurse. In some hospitals, management responsibility may rest with the administrator who heads the medical-surgical unit that houses the rehabilitation service.

Development Concerns: Various restrictions apply to DRG-exempt rehabilitation units. For example, at least 75 percent of patients treated must suffer from one or more of 10 designated conditions during the entire year of a unit's operation. This rule helps ensure that Medicare reimbursement will fund only those patients whose conditions can be best aided by rehabilitation services. In addition, HCFA established this rule to discourage hospitals from converting beds from acute care to rehabilitation and back again whenever doing so would capture additional revenues. If a hospital is adding new rehabilitation beds and converting some acute beds, no more than 50 percent of the beds in the resulting rehabilitation unit may be converted beds; at least half of the beds must be newly licensed.

Regional HCFA offices can supply details on these and other regulations.

Most hospitals with inpatient Medicare rehabilitation units also offer outpatient rehabilitation services, as well as programs designed to restore function to younger persons. It is not unusual for a hospital to have a distinct part Medicare unit and a general rehabilitation department located in different areas. Staff usually will overlap to some extent, particularly the special therapists. An outpatient program will receive many patients from the inpatient program. Hospitals should take these interactions into account when developing DRG-exempt rehabilitation units.

A review process must precede Medicare reimbursement, but this need not be conducted by a government agency. The Commission on Accreditation of Rehabilitation Facilities (CARF) is a not-for-profit organization with "deemed status," meaning that their accreditation is accepted for reimbursement purposes in lieu of Medicare review. (HCFA may nevertheless make revisits to inspect a facility.) Unlike the Medicare process, a CARF review involves rehabilitation professionals whose primary responsibilities are to other full-time jobs within the field. The cost for a CARF review is $550 per person per day plus a $350 application fee; at an average of two persons for two days, the total charge is $2550. Although this is more expensive than a Medicare review, the CARF process is consultative as well as evaluative, providing a hospital with expert input from two rehabilitation professionals.

Information Sources: The American Hospital Association's Section for Rehabilitation Hospitals and Programs offers a wealth of information about hospital-based rehabilitation services. Contact this organization at 840 North Lake Shore Drive, Chicago, IL 60611; (312) 280-6671.

Another source of information is the Commission on Accreditation of Rehabilitation Facilities, 2500 North Pantano Road, Tucson, AZ 85715; (602) 886-8575.

A third source is the National Association of Rehabilitation Facilities in McLean, Virginia. Their mailing address and phone number are P.O. Box 17675, Washington, DC 20041; (703) 556-8848.

Respite Care

Family and friends of the impaired elderly spend a great deal of time and energy providing support and care. In many cases, this involves a round-the-clock commitment for direct care or preventive supervision. In order to relieve primary caregivers of the pressure of unyielding responsibility, some hospitals offer respite programs. Respite care is short-term, temporary care provided to offer relief to the primary caregivers of impaired elderly individuals.

Like hospice care, *respite* is more a concept than a place. Respite care can be delivered in a hospital, nursing home, board and care facility, or in the elderly person's home. Care may last for several hours or several days, sometimes extending for a week or more. Unskilled staff or even volunteers may provide care.

Respite care can be incorporated into existing home health care, adult day care, or general inpatient programs. Thus, a hospital may find that the establishment and management of a respite care program may require less additional effort than other types of programs. A day-only home care operation may need to extend its hours to include round-the-clock coverage, and an adult day care program would have to add an overnight inpatient component. For inpatient respite care, staff sensitivity training is desirable. Marketing will involve a somewhat different focus, and reimbursement patterns will vary. However, most hospitals find that respite care programs do not require the wholesale importing of new skills that are essential to many other elder services.

Value: Respite care is extremely beneficial to the patient's family. Surveys of community attitudes pertaining to long-term care frequently reveal the need for relief felt by many caregivers who are unable to leave their elderly relative or friend unattended. Respite care, whether for a day or a month, allows caregivers rest, vacation, or simply a chance to attend to matters requiring time away from home.

Because of the tremendous need for respite care, hospitals generate a great deal of goodwill by providing such care. A respite care program is also an excellent direct marketing tool. The patient who is well treated during respite care is all the more likely to use the sponsoring hospital in the future, and caregivers also are predisposed to visit for their own health care needs.

Although little third-party funding is available to cover the costs of respite care, a hospital nonetheless may reap financial benefits from offering a program. Private-pay programs, whether facility- or home-based, often turn a profit. Inpatient programs may allow hospitals to generate revenue from otherwise empty acute care beds. Demand for ancillary services usually increases somewhat. For other types of programs, adding a respite care component to home health care or adult day care programs may broaden their appeal and generate additional revenues.

Cost: The cost of a respite care program depends largely on its form. At the high end of the spectrum are the capital costs for constructing a new facility. Construction costs can easily run into the millions of dollars. Another option involves renovating a nearby residential facility, which typically costs from $50,000 to $250,000. At the low end, converting acute inpatient beds or expanding a home health care or adult day care program to offer respite care involves few or no capital expenditures.

Operating costs for bedded programs outside of the hospital are similar to those of intermediate care facilities and primarily involve labor expenses. Inpatient respite care programs generate relatively small marginal costs, often in the $5 to $10 per day range. For home-based programs, operating costs are extensions of those incurred for daytime services.

Staffing: Staffing needs for respite care depend on the program's size and nature. A bedded unit must have a registered nurse available on a 24-hour basis; other staffing will be similar to that of an intermediate care facility, with LPNs and aides providing most of the care. A geriatrician usually will be employed on a part-time basis. Home-based programs predominantly are staffed by aides and LPNs. Some additional sensitivity training—regarding special physical, mental, and perceptual needs of the elderly—is desirable for staff who are to work with respite care guests.

Revenues: Nearly all respite care revenues come from individuals and their families; little third-party reimbursement currently is available. In practice, Medicare or private insurance may cover brief respite care as a portion of home health care services, but no such coverage is possible for overnight or longer care. In 1989, the Medicare program will pay for up to 80 hours annually of respite care provided by a home health agency. The benefit was added by the catastrophic coverage law. To be eligible, the chronically ill person must be dependent on a voluntary caregiver to perform two activities of daily living, and must have met either the Part B catastrophic limit of $1370 for copayments and deductibles or the $600 prescription drug deductible for the year (see HCFA Fact Sheet on Catastrophic Health Insurance).

Typical daily rates for respite care are similar to those of area hotels, usually in the $50 to $80 range. This can generate significant, if not substantial, revenues for sponsoring hospitals. For example, North Penn Hospital in Lansdale, Pennsylvania, garnered over $100,000 during the first two years of its inpatient respite care program at relatively little additional cost.

Market: The users of respite care are the frail, dependent elderly. Most administrators initially are surprised at the disability levels of many guests, and some programs screen out the more severely functionally impaired. It is not unusual for half or more of a program's guests to suffer from Alzheimer's disease. Guests with no mental disabilities often are quite frail physically.

Although older adults are the users of respite care, the most frequent purchasers and decision-makers are the families of disabled older persons. Thus, the primary market for respite care services is comprised of the adult children and middle-aged relatives of older adults who are unable or unwilling to be left alone. This is a difficult segment to identify. Members of caregiver support groups are obvious candidates, but represent only a fraction of the market. Some potential guests or their families use the hospital at some point each year, but many do not.

Physicians also represent an important market segment. Most potential respite care guests visit one or more physicians during the course of a year, usually with a caregiver. Doctors and their staffs are in a good position to recognize the need for respite services and recommend a suitable program.

Marketing: A respite setting that most resembles a hotel has the best chance of success. Many caregivers who leave their older relatives during an out-of-town vacation feel some guilt, which might be assuaged by a hospital providing deluxe accommodations for the guest. Attractive surroundings also make it more beneficial for the sponsoring hospital to invite potential guests and their families to explore the facility in advance of a stay.

Due to the difficulty of identifying and targeting decision-makers for respite services, most programs use a broad advertising approach. Print, radio, and television ads have been used, with newspaper advertising being the most widespread approach. Some programs have found radio to be the most effective medium. In any case, advertising should be stepped up during the months preceding vacation seasons, especially summer, since a primary reason for using respite services is to allow a family to leave town for vacation.

Caregiver support groups are fertile ground for marketing respite care services. They can be contacted personally or through mailings. Adult day care programs are likely to serve many elders who might use respite facilities, and both day care patients and their families should be targeted. The same is true for senior centers and other places where elders gather regularly.

Some programs use attractive posters or brochures to promote their services. These may be sent to physicians to display in their offices, or to senior centers and organizations. Other individuals who might recommend respite care programs and should be contacted include clergy, bank trust officers, and human resource managers of local businesses.

Competition: Because relatively few respite care services are available at this point, competition is not a major issue for most programs. Hospitals offering respite services in an inpatient or free-standing setting are unlikely to feel much competition from home care programs, as the latter tend to be used for very short durations, usually less than 24 hours. Nursing homes or adult day care centers that add overnight services could offer more competition.

Hospitals have several advantages over other types of respite care providers. Community members tend to have high levels of confidence in hospitals and feel secure leaving town knowing that their loved ones are in a safe environment with medical attention readily available. Hospitals also have marketing advantages, since many potential guests or their caregivers pass through the institution at some point. The medical staff is another hospital resource that can be drawn upon to refer guests.

Hospitals may also have some disadvantages in comparison to other respite care providers. Hospital-based programs tend to staff their programs at higher levels, increasing their costs. Social service agencies with their own respite programs may have greater exposure than hospitals to chronic, long-term care patients who may be potential guests. The same is true for nursing homes and adult day care programs with respite services. Hospitals with older or more traditional facilities that do not in any way resemble hotels may be less appealing to guests and their families, although the same is likely to hold for adult day care centers or nursing homes. In any case, due to the dearth of respite care programs in most communities, most hospital-sponsored respite services currently are not threatened by competition.

Timetable: Programs requiring facility construction or renovation may require a year or so to develop. Other respite care programs can be established in a matter of months. Planning, which was time consuming for early programs, can be completed more quickly using existing services as models. Some degree of premarketing is necessary: public advertising and notifying the medical staff, local providers, and the aging network of upcoming services should start weeks or even months before the program opens.

Staff training also must be conducted in advance, but this usually can be completed in a few days. Many services add such components as an exit interview with the family or an extensive health assessment after the program is introduced. Overall, a respite care program, especially one based in an inpatient unit, may be established relatively quickly.

Management: Hospitals possess the management skills necessary to operate either an inpatient or freestanding respite care program. Most inpatient programs are concentrated in one area of a hospital rather than spread throughout the institution. Typically, an inpatient respite service will be managed by the unit administrator for the floor housing the program. A freestanding respite care center often is the responsibility of the hospital's director of eldercare services.

Development Concerns: Many respite care programs include medical services as a standard aspect of any stay. These may involve a comprehensive assessment upon entry, a follow-up care plan written by the nursing staff, and daily physician visits. Such services add only marginally to program costs.

Most respite care programs screen out the severely disabled elderly, preferring to serve only the mildly or moderately functionally impaired. Some programs, especially those located off an inpatient unit with limited capacity, limit length of stay to 60 or 90 days. Length of stay generally averages between 5 and 15 days, depending on the community and the type of program.

Respite care dovetails well with other eldercare services. Health assessment capabilities can be added to the beginning of a respite stay. Older persons using an adult day care or Alzheimer's treatment center may be potential guests. A home care or skilled or intermediate nursing care program can be modified to include a respite component. Families of the frail elderly using hospital-sponsored caregiver support groups or aging resource centers may be very interested in respite services for their relatives.

Information Sources: Because respite care is a relatively new service, there are few central information sources about the field. North Penn Hospital in Lansdale, Pennsylvania, is an excellent source of information regarding setting up a respite program. For information, contact the Administrator of Marketing and Public Affairs, North Penn Hospital, 100 Medical Campus Drive, Lansdale, PA 19446; (215) 368-2100.

For background information, Project SHARE in Rockville, Maryland, has published *A How-to Manual on Providing Respite Care for Family Caregivers.* The manual can be ordered for $13.95 from Project SHARE, P.O. Box 2309, Rockville, MD 20852, or by calling (301) 231-9539. Project SHARE prefers requests be made in writing with prepayment included.

Children of Aging Parents, Inc., publishes a "starter packet" for $22 to assist caregivers in establishing self-help support groups. Children of Aging Parents may be contacted at (215) 945-6900.

Congregate Residential Communities

The variety of congregate housing options for the elderly has spawned a welter of labels that are inconsistently applied. This has caused much confusion among both the public and the retirement industry. Elderly housing facilities vary in terms of living options and proximity of nursing care, but perhaps the most salient distinction among the various options involves the degree of financial commitment required.

In *basic congregate care*, elderly persons rent their own apartments on a monthly basis and share most meals; there is no entry fee. Traditionally, many such facilities have been subsidized by government funds directed at the low-income elderly. Nursing care generally is not included in the arrangement, although many congregate housing communities are sponsored by and located near hospitals. A professional staff person is available to administer services and social activities.

Continuing care residential communities are a type of congregate residential community that offer nursing facilities on or near the premises. The most common financial arrangements involve substantial entry fees and rental agreements guaranteeing lifetime occupancy; there may or may not be a monthly fee. Often the CCRC campus includes three levels of housing offering a continuum of care assistance: independent living apartments, personal care units, and a skilled nursing facility. Some communities allow tenants to purchase their apartments.

A *life care community* is a type of CCRC with an initial entrance fee that entitles an individual to long-term care for life. Typically, skilled nursing care is available on the campus, although some facilities instead have arrangements with local nursing homes.

This section will focus on CCRCs, either with or without life care components. These facilities also are known generically as *retirement communities* or *retirement centers*.

An increasing variety of retirement housing opportunities are available to the elderly. While publicly sponsored housing complexes have existed for years, private residential housing communities with long-term care facilities on site are largely a phenomenon of the 1980s. Because definitions vary and no national registry exists, there are no precise statistics on the number of CCRCs nationwide. Recent estimates by the American Association of Homes for the Aged (AAHA) put the total at between 683 and 700 in 1987, up from approximately 100 in 1979. The AAHA's conservative estimate is for 50 new continuing care retirement communities per year in the near term, growing to an annual rate of 125 by the year 2000. A 1986 *Modern Healthcare* survey reported that in 1985, 13 congregate care centers were completed and 80 new centers were planned.

Similarly, 15 life care centers were completed in 1985 and 67 were planned.

The majority of CCRCs are freestanding rather than hospital-based, although hospitals are entering the field in increasing numbers. The *Modern Healthcare* survey found that of facilities planned, started, or completed during 1985, nearly one-fourth of congregate care centers and almost one-third of life care centers were hospital-affiliated. The vast majority—over 95 percent—of facilities are owned by not-for-profit and religious organizations; as of mid-1986, there were only about a dozen proprietary CCRCs in the nation. Multiunit hospital systems owned or leased 100 centers in 1987, up 20.5 percent from 83 in 1986. Nine multiunit hospital systems managed 43 centers, up 87 percent from 23 in 1986. Nursing home chains operated 216 retirement centers in 1987, up 8.5 percent from 199 in 1986. Manor Care entered the market in 1987 with a fee-for-service health care arrangement. National Medical Enterprises, which owns the Hillhaven nursing home chain, is one of the largest proprietary operators, with 12 units in 1987.

However, profit-seeking entrepreneurs and chains are entering the field. Marriott Corporation, the hotel and restaurant firm, is planning to build several life care retirement centers during the next few years. Sears, one of the nation's largest retailers, is also entering the field through its freestanding company, Mature Outlook. The Forum Group, a developer of life care communities, was ranked first by *Inc.* magazine on its list of fastest growing publicly held American companies.

Continuing care retirement centers offer a broad array of services. All offer housing and meals (one to three congregate meals daily). Laundry, transportation, and maid or homemaker chore assistance usually are available. Most retirement centers offer nursing services, which may be contracted out to a nearby nursing home or provided on the premises, and about half provide personal care services. There is usually some form of emergency medical response system offered. Retirement centers commonly offer social and recreational facilities, including common areas and exercise rooms. Although hospital care generally is not provided, residents are guaranteed that they can return to the community following hospitalization.

The majority of CCRCs provide free transportation for their residents to frequently visited local points. Shopping centers, hospitals, senior centers, and libraries are common destinations for a retirement community's free transportation services.

Value: Retirement centers are designed to encourage residents to live as independently as possible for as long as possible. By entering a congregate community, the elderly enjoy enhanced social contact and supportive services. Centers with a medical component also assure older persons of long-term care services; in life care centers, these services usually are provided at no additional charge. By allowing an individual to choose a long-term care system before services are needed, life care communities increase a person's sense of control over his or her future. Additionally, the concentration of several services into one community enables the resident to remain in a familiar environment when new services are needed, eliminating the trauma typically associated with moving.

A hospital benefits in several regards from being affiliated with a retirement center. First, such a facility can generate a great deal of revenue. A 1987 survey of 173 retirement centers by the accounting firm of Laventhol & Horwath found that median entrance fees ranged from approximately $25,000 to $75,000, depending on the apartment's size and the type of facility; median monthly fees varied from about $600 to $800. A study by AAHA found the average entry fee for one person to be $45,300 and the monthly fee $715; for two persons the fees averaged $65,000 yearly and $808 monthly. A 200-bed facility could generate monthly fees of $150,000, or $1.8 million a year; if turnover averaged 11.5 percent annually, revenues from entrance fees would add nearly a million dollars more once the facility had matured.

Most CCRCs generate a surplus of revenues over expenses for their not-for-profit owners. Although poor planning and unexpectedly high nursing care utilization have driven several life care centers into bankruptcy, numerous institutions have demonstrated that a well-planned and well-managed retirement center can be profitable. The up-front cash inflow for CCRCs is high, and once turnover begins to occur regularly (after 7 to 15 years), typical rates of return are in the range of 15 to 20 percent. However, CCRCs rarely provide a quick financial return. Hospitals and others considering entering the CCRC market should be prepared to sustain losses in the first few years.

A second value of a retirement center is that a hospital can discharge frail elderly patients without hesitation because of the additional support available in the center. In addition, a life care or congregate care community can be an effective means by which to attract potential inpatients. Residents needing acute care services are more likely to enter the sponsoring hospital, if it is properly marketed: about 55 percent of the residents of Methodist Retirement Center in Madison, Wisconsin, choose the sponsoring Methodist Hospital and its medical staff for health care.

Residents of a CCRC may benefit a hospital in other ways. Almost half of the volunteer service hours contributed to Methodist Hospital are logged by residents of the affiliated retirement center. A retirement facility also allows a hospital to extend its service area by attracting elderly persons from nearby communities. Finally, unlike nursing homes, retirement centers are marketed to persons who are relatively healthy and who generally have the financial wherewithal to pay for services. This is an ideal population to have living within a hospital's service area.

Cost: Capital costs of constructing a retirement center range from $10 million to $100 million, depending on the number of structures involved (e.g., apartments, skilled nursing facilities) and the amenities included. Marriott expects to spend $40 million to $70 million on each 250- to 350-bed life care center. Typical capital costs for existing CCRCs range from $25 million to $40 million, but the median costs are rising quickly as facilities become increasingly upscale.

Operating costs vary by type of facility. Centers that are oriented toward nursing care tend to have higher labor costs than those oriented primarily toward retirement, with the exception of salaries for nursing personnel. The distinction between orientations is based on a ration of apartments to nursing beds in a community; all facilities considered have some nursing beds. Overall, a typical 200-apartment community with a 60-bed nursing unit and a 25-bed personal care center would pay gross salaries of approximately $1.25 million. The Laventhol & Horwath survey found that centers oriented toward retirement spend twice as much on food management per meal as those oriented toward nursing care (18 cents versus 9 cents), but only a third as much on medical care ($319 versus $889). These differences reflect both the priorities of the communities and the needs and preferences of the individuals attracted to them. Marketing costs per unit averaged about $2750 in 1984, or just over $500,000 for a typical facility.

Staffing: A typical retirement community with apartments housing 200 residents, a 60-bed nursing center, and a 25-bed personal care unit has approximately 100 employees, although this figure may range from 40 to over 250, depending largely on the number of residents. A community primarily oriented toward nursing will be staffed at higher levels. Nursing-oriented facilities have higher nursing staff ratios, averaging 40 FTEs versus 26 for retirement-oriented facilities. Although the average number of apartments in such communities is lower, the care needs of their residents are greater. Nursing-oriented facilities have a median staff of 120, but some large centers will employ as many as 400.

Nursing staff, including nursing administrators and an administrator for the nursing center itself, account for the largest share of employees in both types of communities, but the proportion is greater for centers oriented toward nursing care. Dietary, housekeeping, and laundry staff also account for a large number of employees. These latter groups are among the lowest paid workers in retirement communities.

Revenues: Currently, this is a private-pay market. Medicare and private health insurance rarely pay for services provided by a retirement center. With entrance fees of at least $10,000 and monthly rental rates generally exceeding $500, individuals qualifying for Medicaid or other income-based entitlements are unlikely to be able to enter a retirement community. However, the Laventhol & Horwath survey found that 10 percent of residents of retirement-oriented (as opposed to nursing-oriented) centers might eventually require financial assistance, and that about 5.5 percent presently required aid. In those cases, the centers either drew money from contingency funds set up for that purpose or used current operating funds.

Most residents finance entrance into CCRCs through the sale of their houses. This option is made more attractive to the elderly by federal law, which permits a one-time, tax-free capital gain on up to $125,000 earned from the sale of a home. Since about 62 percent of older Americans currently own their homes free and clear, many persons over age 65 are well within financial striking distance of entering a retirement community.

Retirement centers vary in their financial arrangements with residents. Life care centers usually charge a substantial entrance fee plus monthly rental payments; these fees guarantee admission into and payment for a nursing facility if necessary. Pay-in-full contracts require a large entrance fee that covers all future expenses; no additional monthly or long-term care charges are assessed. Some or all of the entrance fee usually is refundable if the resident leaves the community within the first few years. Some life care centers refund the fee whenever the resident leaves and even return the full amount to the individual's estate upon death.

Turn-over-assets contracts require entrants to sign over all financial assets to the center in exchange for lifetime care. Other agreements do not include nursing care with the entrance fee, but guarantee admission into the facility when needed; care is provided on a fee-for-service basis. Recently, there has been a movement away from all-inclusive lump-sum payments entitling residents to full care for life. Rapidly increasing life expectancy has confounded actuarial assumptions, causing turnover to be lower than expected and decreasing revenue from entrance fees; thus life care center owners are seeking to reduce their risk of providing long-term care over long periods of time. Many new facilities are avoiding the risks of life care, opting instead for a congregate care arrangement involving monthly rental but no entry fee; nursing care is not included and often not available onsite. Other new facilities tend to have more nursing home beds in recognition of the aging-in-place phenomenon.

In most cases, entrance or monthly rental fees do not cover acute care, although Medicare and Medigap insurance tend to cover such services, just as they do for nonresidents. However, a growing number of retirement centers offer prepaid health plans that cover hospital and physician services as well as services ranging from prescription drugs to eyeglasses. Hospital-based retirement communities in particular are interested in such policies as avenues to channel patients into their acute care beds. A concept that is gaining momentum in the industry is that of offering long-term care insurance as part of the purchase package. National Medical Enterprises is developing a complex in Massachusetts that will offer an insurance package through Metropolitan Life Insurance Company, New York.

Market: The market for retirement centers consists of relatively affluent men and women usually over age 62. The majority of persons entering CCRCs are between the ages of 75 and 84. The Laventhol & Horwath survey of the life care retirement center industry reported that residents' average age at entry in 1987 was 78 for both men and women entering retirement-oriented facilities and 79 for men and women entering nursing-oriented facilities. The average age of all residents was 82. These figures increased significantly—by one to two years each—since the previous year. Between 75 and 78 percent of retirement center residents are female. Over the years 1984 to 1986, there was a slight increase in the percentage of men in these facilities.

Most retirement center residents come from the surrounding community. A 50-mile radius defines a maximum market area. On average, approximately 80 percent of residents enter the facility from a community within 25 miles of the center; one-third come from within a 10-mile radius. These figures vary with the orientation of the facility, the proximity to competitors, and the population density. Some retirement centers get 90 percent of their residents from their 25-mile radius primary market area.

As with elderly persons who do not live in retirement centers, a substantial proportion of CCRC residents live near one or more of their children. Approximately half of all residents live within a 30-minute drive of at least one of their children; this figure is slightly larger for residents of nursing-oriented centers and those in suburban or rural areas as opposed to cities.

Marketing: The CCRC market offers a wealth of opportunity. The American Hospital Association reports that continuing care and life care communities are the least available long-term care services offered by hospitals. Demand for retirement centers is high in many areas, and it is not uncommon for there to be waiting lists. Older facilities tend to have longer waiting lists than newer ones, perhaps because they are better known in the surrounding communities. The Laventhol & Horwath survey found that waitlists averaged 15 months for a one-bedroom apartment in facilities built prior to 1975, and 8 months for newer units. For two-bedroom apartments the wait averaged 30 months for older centers and 15 months for newer ones. With all of the recent activity in the field however, some metropolitan areas, such as San Diego, are becoming overbuilt, according to industry analysts.

The marketing of CCRCs is often intense, as management focuses on attracting the high end of the market. Promotion for a retirement center can and should begin well in advance of its construction. Marketers find that it is difficult to persuade elderly persons to give up their homes, leave their neighborhoods, and move into retirement centers, even though the geographic shift usually is minor. A retirement community should aim to have at least half of its apartments rented before it is ready for residents to move in.

Pricing is a key element of the marketing plan. Careful market research is crucial in determining both price levels and payment type. Prices must be set with an eye to competitors and to area home equity levels, which will to some extent determine how much people will be capable of paying. Research must investigate attitudes toward acute and long-term health care to determine whether demand is greater for a life care concept, a congregate care community with fee-for-service nursing care, a prepaid all-inclusive package, or some other arrangement. Market research should also determine whether prospective residents prefer to purchase, rent, or lease their apartments, and what effect the refundability of the deductible will have on demand. The current industry trend is away from all inclusive contracts toward fee-for-service arrangements.

The location of a retirement center is a critical marketing decision. Choosing a safe, secure site is essential. Other issues include physical attractiveness, geographic position within the primary market, and access to mass transportation. Also important are proximity to health care providers, banks, shops, senior centers, religious institutions, and retail stores. Due to the broad range of preferences regarding these options, local market research should be employed to shed light on what elements potential customers view as most desirable.

Proper siting of a retirement center can also aid future marketing efforts by providing a convenient spot for nonresident seniors to meet. Retirement centers are wise to offer their facilities generously to community groups concerned with issues regarding the elderly; a central location makes such offers more appealing. Congregate living communities themselves may sponsor meetings on topics of interest to older persons, thus serving the dual purpose of providing community education and introducing prospective residents to their campuses. Some CCRCs are considering establishing aging resource centers open to the local community, both as a service to residents and as a means to draw other older persons to the center.

Although individuals enter retirement centers in part for reasons of financial and life security, they are usually attracted by the independent life-style available. Promotional advertising should emphasize a commitment to wellness and a healthy life-style, with the notion of security as an additional benefit. Older persons are more likely to respond to a new and exciting living environment than to a place to go to grow old.

Competition: The presence of a competitor within an area need not be bad news for a hospital considering developing a retirement center. As with other relatively new concepts, the first organization in an area to offer a new service must expend substantial resources to educate consumers about that service. Subsequent entrants can spend fewer resources on general education and more on promoting their own facilities.

Retirement centers sponsored by not-for-profit district and religious hospitals have a marketing advantage over proprietary facilities in the eyes of many consumers. Older persons invest a substantial sum of money in the initial fee on the assumption that the sponsor will provide housing and (usually) health care services for the remainder of their lives; institutions affiliated with religious denominations or long-standing community organizations are considered by some to be more reliable and trustworthy than those owned by profit-seeking firms. For similar reasons, hospital-based retirement centers have advantages over freestanding CCRCs.

At present, primary competition for congregate living facilities comes from other hospital-based retirement centers, from freestanding facilities, and, increasingly, from national chains. In addition, CCRCs with a skilled or intermediate nursing home on the campus will compete for patients with other homes in the area. Most CCRCs attempt to draw nursing patients from the surrounding community since initially (and perhaps indefinitely) the nursing home beds will not be filled by residents of the retirement center.

Timetable: A retirement center is a major project requiring a substantial amount of time for researching, planning, developing, building, and marketing. Preliminary market analysis, financial planning, site identification and purchase, financial feasibility determination, and board approval will require at least a year and probably two. Construction itself averages from one to two years, during which time the marketing effort begins.

On average, half of CCRC units are rented within about a year of the start of construction. Typically, by the time the facility has been open for a year, about three-fourths of the apartments are occupied. On average, 95 percent occupancy is reached approximately 18 months after the facility is opened.

Management: There is relatively little transference of skills from the hospital industry to the CCRC field. Congregate housing is a real estate project with a health care component, not the other way around. Consequently, hospitals sponsoring CCRCs nearly always hire consultants and/or developers to design, build, and market the communities. In addition, CCRCs are usually operated as separate corporate entities from a sponsoring hospital. Typically, the facility is managed by the owner rather than by a management company, although the latter situation is not uncommon.

Hospitals may joint-venture with entrepreneurs or developers to build CCRCs, or they may hire the necessary talent. Joint-venturing often has financial advantages, since the capital costs of building are high. A properly structured joint venture may allow hospitals to take advantage of their not-for-profit status to float bonds in order to finance the venture. While new tax legislation reduces the availability of tax-exempt financing, not-for-profit institutions still retain an advantage in this regard.

Development Concerns: Grubb & Ellis Company warns that less than 3 percent of the elderly population will ever by interested in moving into a CCRC, and that there is a possibility of serious short-term oversupply. Whether oversupply becomes a problem depends on what proportion of the many projects presently being considered are ever completed. Laventhol & Horwath estimates that no more than 10 percent of a community's income-qualified elderly are likely to live in some type of congregate housing, depending on the area. The consulting firm Lewin/ICF, based in Washington, D.C., estimates that 2.6 percent of adults between 75 and 84 will desire to live in life care centers in the future, and another 18.1 will seek congregate housing.

Continuing care residential communities should be designed to have enough nursing beds to meet the needs of the mature community. Many states require that a nursing station may supervise no more than 60 beds. Consequently, many CCRCs have exactly that number of nursing beds and, thus, need build only one nursing station. Retirement-oriented centers averaged four apartments per nursing bed in the Laventhol & Horwath survey. For nursing-oriented facilities the ratio is 1.2 apartment units per nursing home bed is 0.9.

Regulation: As the industry matures, more regulations will be introduced. This trend toward regulation has been hastened by reports of several CCRCs going bankrupt and having to be sold. In response to industry needs and public perception, the Continuing Care Accreditation Commission (CCAC) was created. The CCAC is an independent commission established in 1985 and sponsored by the American Association of Homes for the Aging. The CCAC represents a major force in self-regulation of the CCRC industry. The accreditation is based on an academic model using self-assessment of 14 standards. There are currently 52 facilities in 17 states that have received accreditation: 15 of these are in California. Thus far, no proprietary facilities have been accredited, but several have expressed an interest in going through the process in the coming year. The CCAC sees its role as assisting "in the enhancement of the continuing care industry by providing CCRCs with external stimulation for continual self-improvement."

By 1988, 20 states had regulations involving CCRCs, and several others were considering passing legislation pertaining to the industry. Most regulations are designed to protect residents from losing their investments should the retirement center run into financial difficulty. Nearly all states have regulations governing the skilled nursing component of congregate retirement centers, particularly for those receiving some reimbursement from Medicare or Medicaid. Many of the laws require the sale of 50 percent to 60 percent of a facility's units before construction begins, thus minimizing the risk of failure.

Information Sources: The American Association of Homes for the Aged is a good source of information about CCRCs and life care centers. The address is 1129 20th Street, N.W., Suite 400, Washington, DC 20036; (202) 296-5960. The Winklevoss and Powell report, which an AAHA study is designed to update, is published by Richard D. Irwin at 1818 Ridge Road, Homewood, IL 60430; (312) 798-6000.

A relatively new organization is the National Association for Senior Living Industries (NASLI) at 125 Cathedral Street, Annapolis, MD 21401; (301) 263-0991. The NASLI members represent the broad spectrum of individuals and firms involved in senior living. The organization sponsors conferences and site visits around the nation, and publishes monographs on topics of interest to members.

The accounting firm of Laventhol & Horwath has extensive experience in the life care/retirement industry and publishes an annual report. The firm has branches in several cities. Its executive offices are located at 1845 Walnut Street, Philadelphia, PA 19103; (215) 299-1600.

Senior Membership Programs

A senior membership program (SMP) is a bundle of eldercare services. Hospital-based membership programs for older people offer a variety of benefits, ranging from VIP admission for members to discounts at local merchants to free health screenings. From the consumers' perspective, the SMP makes it easier to understand the scope of eldercare services offered by the hospital. It also provides a single point of entry to these services.

For the hospital, the purpose of an SMP is to create loyalty among possible patients. A well-conceived SMP carries great marketing potential: older people who have come to identify with a hospital through its SMP are more likely to use the institution if they require hospitalization. In addition to this primary market, a number of secondary markets exist. For instance, adult children and, in many cases, elderly parents of SMP members, are more inclined to use the hospital, having heard about it from the SMP member.

The SMP is designed to:

- build and maintain consumer loyalty;
- increase utilization of acute care services, thus enhancing market share;

- bundle services into programs that are more easily understood by older people and their families;

- group services in such a way that they can be managed as a product line; and

- create an eldercare identity for the provider.

The scope of SMPs varies widely. Some offer substantial benefits to older people and their families. In these cases, creation of the program itself generates a number of new services which have not previously been offered and which serve a significant need. Such senior membership programs are genuine eldercare programs. At the other end of the spectrum are enrollment programs primarily geared toward promotion. These SMPs bundle together existing services in an attempt to gain market share. Services may be discounted but usually are not well-coordinated. This type of program is more of a marketing strategy than an eldercare program. However, most senior membership programs share some essential characteristics. These include:

- enticements for members to use the sponsoring hospital or medical staff, such as discounted fees and transportation services;

- assistance in navigating the maze of health services and reimbursement, such as Medicare paperwork assistance and flexible payment plans; and

- benefits associated with being a member of a club, such as free parking and accelerated admission.

Each program has its own bundle of benefits to achieve these goals. Typical program benefits include:

- *central telephone number* providing a single point of entry to all eldercare services offered by the institution and staffed by someone trained to be sensitive to the needs of older people and knowledgeable about all programs and services available.

- *health newsletter,* which may be produced inhouse or purchased from a national supplier, containing information about health in general and the sponsoring provider in particular.

- *senior advisor,* available to help members with any of a variety of health and health care problems, who often has a nursing or social services background and may perform various duties, from advising members on insurance policies to counseling families.

- *paperwork and Medicare filing assistance* to help members minimize the frustration and confusion of insurance and Medicare forms. (This is the most popular benefit offered by senior membership programs.)

- *membership card,* to convey a sense of value for the program, identifying members at special events or when they apply for discounts and bonuses, and serves as a reminder of the program and its sponsor. (Membership cards typically are credit card size and range from simple cardboard printed cards to sophisticated plastic cards with the member's medical history on a magnetic strip on the back of the card.)

- *"frequent flyer benefits"* that convey special privileges to members and their families, named after the airlines' reward system for their customers. Typical benefits include free parking at the hospital, a private hospital room at a semiprivate rate, physician referral services, discounts on meals in the hospital cafeteria, discounts in the hospital gift shop, free tea or coffee in the hospital lobby, free telephone and/or television during a hospital stay, flexible payment plans, free or discounted health screening, and accelerated or advance check-in for hospital stays.

Some programs also offer additional benefits, such as free or discounted transportation to and from the medical facility or physician office, free home health care for a few days following hospital discharge, free use of an aging resource center, physician house calls, a free meal in the room for visitors during member's hospitalization, an overnight cot for a relative or friend of a hospitalized member, information and referral services, care management to help individuals use the complicated network of eldercare services, health education classes, nutrition counseling, and social events.

Revenues: Senior membership programs that charge an enrollment fee will recognize some revenues from the program, but these revenues typically do not cover the costs of the program (which are concentrated in salaries and marketing). Most hospital administrators recognize senior membership programs as loss leaders for other services of the hospital. The annual membership fee ($5 to $25) that some programs assess members is designed more to create the appearance of value than to bring in revenue. The payoff from senior membership programs is seen in increased use of the hospital itself and its physicians and services.

Marketing: The age of eligibility for membership programs varies. The most common age breaks are at 65 or 55, although some programs specify 60 or 50. Which age is most appropriate depends on the purpose of the program. Many senior membership programs design their programs to dovetail with the eligibility for Medicare at age 65. This is logical if the purpose of the program is to serve Medicare beneficiaries. However, most programs have two broader goals: to improve service to older people and to assist the provider's business. Both goals are often better served by using an eligibility age lower than 65.

Marketing a senior membership program is an ongoing activity. Although senior membership programs have been in existence for close to a decade, they are still new to many areas. In such areas, a significant portion of the marketing will involve educating the public about the concept as well as the program itself.

Successful marketing strategies generally incorporate ZIP code-specific direct mailings, advertising in the local media and senior publications, open houses, human interest stories in the media, and extensive public speaking to interested groups by members of the senior membership's staff. Depending on the competitiveness of the local environment and the geographic distribution of the target audience, television and radio advertising can be appropriate. In competitive urban and metropolitan areas, a number of programs have found that they pay to have their message broadcast to a much wider audience than is necessary: they find their advertising dollars are better spent with a more carefully targeted medium. On the other hand, senior membership programs located in more rural, less heavily populated areas often find that local television and radio advertising does reach their more widespread target audience. Each market must be carefully researched to receive the most value for advertising and marketing dollars spent.

An individual program within the senior membership program often can serve as a marketing vehicle itself. For instance, a major component of many senior membership programs is a central telephone number. The telephone number provides members and interested callers with a means of getting specific information about the program and its components, referral information, billing assistance, or any of the other services and programs available.

Competition: The competition for senior membership programs comes from other hospitals, whether or not they have senior membership programs. The objective of the program is to increase revenue for the hospital and its physicians. The competition therefore is any program or physician that attracts and keeps patients' loyalty.

In areas where senior membership programs are relatively new the competition tends to be less intense than in metropolitan areas which have many hospitals with well-developed programs. The question to ask when evaluating the competition is how well the programs fulfill their objective of helping their sponsoring institution. A senior membership program with many alleged members may not be adding significantly to the hospital census. Depending on how success is defined, a competing program with many members may or may not be a success. In evaluating enrollment numbers, it should be kept in mind that since most senior membership programs are free, many seniors sign up for more than one program. Their loyalty to the hospital and its providers has not been won.

Timetable: Depending on the build-or-buy decision, it typically takes between four and eighteen months to implement a program. A purchased program will take approximately four to six months to get up and running from the time of purchase. A program designed inhouse will take significantly longer because of the need to conduct and analyze market research, develop a marketing program, create and test marketing materials, develop or purchase a computer tracking system and develop the program itself.

Administrators of many senior membership programs are finding that they continue to develop new program components and refine existing ones as their membership grows and voices its needs and desires.

Development Concerns: A hospital considering a senior membership program is immediately faced with deciding whether to develop its own program inhouse or purchase one of the nationally franchised programs. The build-or-buy decision must take into account the hospital's internal marketing resources, in addition to its expertise in general eldercare issues. Health care providers without a strong inhouse capability to conduct (or contract out for) reliable market research, advertising, and public relations should consider purchasing a program. The competitive environment will also be a factor in the decision.

Other important inhouse capabilities for developing a program include expertise in telemarketing, in mailing list development and management, in computer tracking, and in health education. The time frame available to have the program available to the community also is a determining factor in the build-or-buy decision: less time is required to make a franchised program operational than to build one from the ground up. The availability of funds and staff and the scope of the planned program are crucial factors in deciding which option to take. Purchased programs also can be tailored, in many cases, to meet the individual needs of the hospital and its community.

The key issues boil down to the capabilities of the organization, the relative cost of building versus buying, and the competitive pressures that may require quick implementation.

Information Sources: There are a number of national franchised senior membership programs available.

Baylor Telemanagement Systems has developed a sophisticated information management and tracking system for SMPs. For information, contact the Vice President of Resource Sales, 3201 Worth Street, P.O. Box 26265, Dallas, TX 75226; (800) 999-5460 or, in the Dallas area, (214) 820-2895.

ElderMed America offers a turnkey senior membership program that can be implemented within six to twelve weeks, either in a generic or a customized form. The ElderMed program includes membership management, microcomputer software, a quarterly magazine for members, all advertising development, as well as national and regional discounts. Contact the Executive Vice President, 20500 Nordhoff Road, Chatsworth, CA 91311; (818) 407-2285.

GoldenCare PLUS is a marketing and promotion plan, customized to each hospital's needs. Features include camera-ready art, advertising development and support, instructions for choosing and training advisors, and a slide presentation for attracting prospective members. For information, contact the Manager of GoldenCare PLUS at Saint Francis Medical Center, 530 Northeast Glen Oak Avenue, Peoria, IL 61637; (309) 655-4110.

Silver Advantage is a microcomputer software program designed to evaluate and guide marketing to seniors while providing valuable information to administrators and physicians. By means of a bar code in the senior membership card, the program stores, sorts, and reports on data collected, allowing for accurate and timely tracking. For information, contact the Senior Services Coordinator, 84 Beaumont Drive, Mason City, IA 50401; (515) 424-7241.

Third Age Life National Marketing Services offers a series of instructional manuals on the development and implementation of hospital-based older adult programs. Six manuals detail innovative program planning models; market research, sensitivity training, care coordination, LIFEPASS$^{\text{(TSM)}}$ enrollment program, computer software program, installation and training, and marketing communications. For information, contact the Manager, 3300 Northwest Expressway, Oklahoma City, OK 73112-4481; (405) 949-4035.

VHA National Access is a VHA Enterprise company that provides products and services to enhance and support a network of VHA hospital senior programs. Products available exclusively to VHA hospitals include newsletter copy, education programs, a media access program, and microcomputer software. For additional information, contact the Vice President, 5215 North O'Connor Road, Suite 2000, Irving, TX 75039; (214) 830-0090.

V.I.P. Advantage^{sm} Program is a customized marketing program that enables health care facilities to develop loyalty with and encourage utilization by their senior adult and caregiver audiences. The program incorporates many components, including internal and external environmental assessments, one-year marketing plan, tracking system development, 180 consulting hours and telephone support. For information, contact Ernst & Whinney, 515 South Flower Street, Suite 2900, Los Angeles, CA 90071; (213) 621-1666.

Skilled Nursing Care

The terms "nursing home" and "nursing care" refer to a variety of facilities and services. For the purposes of this report, these terms are defined as follows:

- *Skilled nursing care* involves 24-hour care of such complexity that at least some of it must be delivered by a registered nurse.

- *Intermediate care* does not require the attention of a registered nurse, but still involves assistance—often physical— that is beyond the capability of an infirm individual. Note, however, that the definition for intermediate care will change in 1990 for homes reimbursed by Medicaid. Nursing home reform legislation passed in 1987 requires that intermediate care facilities employ at least one registered nurse for eight hours a day.

- *Custodial care* is similar to intermediate care, but the term usually is applied to care of chronically ill patients who are not expected to improve.

- A *skilled nursing facility* (SNF) is licensed to provide general skilled care. A SNF is likely to house a significant number of patients—perhaps 30 percent of the census or more— who do not require regular skilled care.

- An *intermediate care facility* (ICF) is licensed to provide intermediate level or custodial care, but not skilled care.

- An *intermediate care facility for the mentally retarded* (ICFMR) is licensed to provide care for mentally disordered patients, usually with some degree of RN involvement.

- *Nursing home* is a generic term that technically refers to SNFs, ICFs, and ICFMRs. Some people also include convalescent homes (which need not provide any level of nursing care) within their definitions of nursing homes.

There are 19,100 nursing homes in the country with over 1.6 million beds. An additional 4000 facilities are custodial care homes. Of the 19,100 homes, 76 percent, or 14,400 homes, are certified by Medicare or Medicaid or both; virtually no uncertified homes provide skilled care. Only 24 percent, or 3500 facilities, of all the certified homes were SNF only. Another 5700, or 40 percent, of all certified homes were certified as both an SNF and an ICF. Of the certified homes, 73 percent, or 10,500, were operated for profit; 21 percent, or 3000, were not-for-profit; and 6 percent, or 900 homes, were owned by public institutions. Homes operated by chains are increasing in numbers, from 28 percent of total homes in 1977 to 41 percent of total homes in 1985. The number of hospitals operating long-term care beds also is increasing. The American Hospital Association reported the number of hospitals operating SNF-only beds increased about 8 percent to 979 hospitals in 1986 from 906 in 1985.

Skilled care generally involves nursing and rehabilitative services. Standard personal care and dietary services are also provided by skilled nursing facilities. In addition, since as many as half of nursing home residents may have psychological or emotional disturbances, mental health services usually are an important component of care.

Value: Skilled nursing care provides needed medical and supportive assistance to the patient on a 24-hour basis outside of the usual acute care hospital setting. Skilled nursing care is less expensive than inpatient care because the services delivered are less intensive. Additional benefits for the patient include greater freedom to move around and receive visitors than a hospital offers, and congregate meals and recreational opportunities that enhance social contact.

A hospital benefits in a number of respects from offering skilled care. As prospective payment encourages hospitals to discharge patients as early as possible, ownership of a skilled care facility increases the availability of skilled care beds for the sponsoring institution. This both prevents the hospital from losing money on a patient ready for discharge but for whom no bed can be found, and allows the capture of additional revenue. A hospital also reaps referral benefits by having a nursing home within its continuum of care, since many patients are discharged from a SNF to a hospital or to their homes with home care support; hospital-based nursing homes can influence the referral choices.

Cost: The capital costs for a skilled nursing facility depend on the method of development. Building a nursing home is often—but not always—the most expensive option. The ballpark construction cost figure that the American Health Care Association uses is $25,000 per bed, but this will vary with facility characteristics and prevailing local construction costs. Buying a SNF tends to be less expensive, with per-bed prices typically falling within the range of $19,000 to $23,000, depending on where the homes are located. The acquisition costs of SNFs recently saw a decrease when the giant nursing home chains, such as Beverly Enterprises, ended years of expansion and began divesting facilities.

Regulations limiting nursing home construction drive prices higher than building costs in many areas. Homes with more than three- and four-bedroom units are worth slightly less due to their lower appeal for private-pay patients. Converting an acute hospital unit or wing to long-term skilled care is the least expensive option, although structural modifications may run as high as $15,000 to $20,000 per bed. Capital or property-related costs typically account for 10 to 15 percent of a facility's total costs.

Patient care costs typically range from $35 to $80 per patient-day. However, extremely needy patients, such as those on respirators, may cost $600 or more per day; earlier discharges resulting from prospective payment incentives are leading to larger numbers of such patients in skilled nursing facilities. Staff-to-patient ratios are an important cost factor, since labor usually accounts for 60 to 70 percent of a skilled nursing care budget. Administrative and general costs typically account for 25 to 30 percent of a SNF's total costs.

Nursing homes report rising labor costs due to the nursing shortage. In a recent survey by the American Health Care Association, 50 percent of responding facilities indicated either a moderate or severe shortage for all types of nursing staff. Nursing homes are unable to compete with the higher salaries nurses are paid by hospitals. The median hourly salary for a general duty RN was $9.92 in a nursing home versus $14.41 in a hospital, according to AHCA. Licensed practical nurses received $7.85 per hour in a nursing home versus $8.74 in a hospital, and nurse assistants received $4.57 in a nursing home versus $6.82 in a hospital. To fill vacancies some nursing homes are relying on temporary help or increasing salaries. Both strategies increase labor costs.

Staffing: A 1983 Iowa study found that staffing levels average eight staff persons per shift at for-profit nursing homes and 11 per shift at not-for-profit homes. Many states regulate staffing levels; California, for instance, requires 2.8 hours of staffing per patient-day for skilled nursing care. The HCFA reports that hospital-based SNFs average 3.9 hours of nursing care per patient-day, while free-standing facilities average 3.27 hours. Urban SNFs average higher staffing ratios than rural facilities. Over 90 percent of hospital-based SNFs have staffing ratios of one nurse to nine beds or less.

The National Center for Health Statistics reports that the average 100-bed nursing home employs 43.4 full-time equivalents providing nursing and personal care. The 100-bed home employs an additional 28 FTEs—5.5 in administration and 22.5 for nonnursing services. Public institutions and not-for-profit homes employ more nurses than average—51.6 FTEs and 47.2 FTEs, respectively, at 100-bed facilities. For-profit homes employ 41.1 nursing FTEs at a 100-bed home.

Just under half of all nurses in hospital-based homes are RNs. Overall, the vast majority of care provided in long-term care facilities is administered by untrained aides and orderlies. This has ramifications for care quality: low pay, lack of job satisfaction, and minimal opportunity for career advancement contribute to a turnover rate approaching 100 percent annually for unskilled long-term care staff. Many nursing home administrators cite staff turnover as a major management challenge.

Certified SNFs hire a significantly greater number of RNs than other certified facilities. The SNFs employed 7.1 RNs per 100 beds, whereas the ICFs employed 2.7 RNs per 100 beds, according to the 1985 National Nursing Home Survey.

Staffing ratios, particularly at ICFs, will change as a result of the Omnibus Budget Reconciliation Act of 1987. As of October 1, 1990 the law requires all certified nursing homes to maintain round-the-clock licensed practical nursing care. Currently, only certified SNFs have been required to provide 24-hour licensed nursing care (provided by either LVNs or LPNs). In addition, the law requires that as of October, 1990, at least one registered nurse be on duty for eight hours a day. The ICFs had been allowed to employ either an RN or an LPN or an LVN during the day shift. The law also requires mandatory training for all current and future nurses aides, full-time social workers in facilities with more than 120 beds, and qualified activities directors and dieticians in all nursing homes.

Skilled nursing facilities generally are staffed by an administrator, a nursing staff, and some number of social workers, dieticians, and aides. Speech, occupational, and vocational therapists are brought in as needed. Volunteers may comprise a portion of a nursing home's staff.

Revenues: On a national level, just over half of the $38 billion spent on nursing home care in 1986 was paid for by patients, families and other private pay sources. About 41 percent of payments are from Medicaid, and only small amounts come from Medicare (1.6 percent) or private insurance (0.8 percent).

Medicaid pays for skilled nursing care in a SNF that is provided on a daily basis by professional or technical personnel. Medicaid also pays for intermediate care provided in an ICF. Although federal regulations are quite specific about the distinctions between skilled and intermediate care, states vary greatly in their use of these levels of care. States such as California and Connecticut have primarily skilled care, while Iowa, Oklahoma, and others consider nearly all the care they provide to be intermediate care. Because Medicaid eligibility is based on a lack of financial resources, reimbursement is only available to the poor or to private-pay patients who have spent down to eligibility levels. This is a common occurrence. In October 1987, the House Select Committee on Aging reported seven in ten single nursing home residents spend down to the federal poverty level after 13 weeks. Within one year, 90 percent face impoverishment.

Medicaid rates vary widely by state. The Institute for Health and

Aging in San Francisco recently tabulated state-by-state SNF and ICF rates between 1984 and 1986. In 1986, SNF rates ranged from $32.16 per day in Arkansas to $152.78 in Alaska. The median daily rate was $50.81. The ICF rates for 1986 varied from a low of $28.14 in Louisiana to $152.18 in Alaska. The median daily rate was $42.54. The variance in rates is partly due to the differences in ancillary services covered by the state. Alaska covers drugs, physical and occupational therapy, and durable medical equipment and other supplies for SNF and ICF residents. Other states only cover some of these ancillary services.

The catastrophic health insurance coverage legislation, enacted into law in 1988, extended the number of skilled days covered by Medicare and applied the copayments to the first eight days of an SNF stay rather than later in the stay. As of January 1989, Medicare pays for up to 150 days of skilled (but not intermediate) care within a benefit period, with a copayment of $20.50 (in 1989) for the first eight days of skilled nursing facility care. The law eliminated a requirement that a beneficiary had to be hospitalized for at least three days prior to admission to a skilled nursing facility. (A benefit period starts the day a person is admitted to a nursing home and ends 60 days after discharge.) Although Medicare covers up to 150 days of skilled care within a benefit period, on average, Medicare paid for only 22 days of nursing care per admission in 1986. In 1987, skilled nursing facilities located within metropolitan statistical areas and affiliated with hospitals received a base rate of $94.21 per patient-day for routine care, compared with $61.41 for freestanding institutions.

The private-pay market has surpassed Medicaid in recent years as the primary source of nursing home revenues. The average price per day is $61 for SNFs and $48 for ICFs. Depending on the local market conditions and beds per room, these costs may be a third again as high. This premium over average Medicaid rates has led to preferential admission of private-pay patients in many areas, exacerbating the placement problem for Medicaid recipients in need of skilled nursing care. However, some states have passed or are considering legislation to limit this practice. Ohio, for example, requires at least 35 percent of all nursing home patients to be Medicaid recipients. And, in 1987, Virginia and California passed legislation prohibiting nursing homes from requiring a guaranteed private fee as a condition for admittance.

While private long-term care insurance pays for only a fraction of nursing home care, the industry is burgeoning. However, the quality of the policies and their value to policyholders needs careful scrutiny. A recent study by a Washington consumer group, United Seniors Health Cooperative, analyzed 77 long-term care policies sold by 21 companies. The policies paid a daily rate ranging from $40 to $100; the most common rate was $50. The covered period was between two to six years. However, only 39 percent of the policyholders would ever collect any benefits, the group found. The remaining 61 percent would be unable to collect because of policy restrictions such as a prior hospitalization requirement for skilled care. Less than half of all nursing home admissions follow hospitalization. Nevertheless, some industry observers predict that long-term care insurance will become a significant contributor to nursing home revenues by the end of the decade.

Employer interest to sponsor long-term care benefits for employees and retirees is increasing. A Washington Business Group on Health survey found that of 147 respondents, 38 percent are investigating the possibility of offering long-term care insurance, and an additional 26 percent plan to do so within the next two years.

Market: Eighty-eight percent, or 1.3 million people, of nursing home residents are over age 65. About 5 percent of elderly persons are in a nursing home at any given time, and one-fifth will receive institutionalized skilled care at some point. The median age at entry for nursing home residents is 80 and climbing; the median age of residents is 84. The primary market for skilled nursing care consists of persons over age 75, who account for four-fifths of current nursing home residents. Residents aged 85 years and older represent 45 percent of the nursing home population; residents between the ages of 75 and 84 account for 39 percent of the group, and residents aged 65 to 74 comprise only 16 percent of the nursing home population.

The nursing home population is disproportionately female and single. Approximately three-fourths of the nursing home population is female. Of women over 75, 76 percent do not have spouses, while for men in that age category only 31 percent do not have spouses.

On average, female residents are older than male residents (84 versus 81 years). The preponderance of elderly women without spousal support often leaves institutional care as the only option.

Cardiovascular disease is the most common diagnosis at the time of admission to a nursing home. Over 30 percent of all nursing home residents have a diagnosis tied to the circulatory system. Mental disorders are the second most common diagnosis, accounting for about 21 percent of admissions. Alzheimer's disease and a few other degenerative brain disorders represent almost 3 percent of the admissions. However, these figures are based on all types of nursing facilities. For SNFs, it is likely that cardiovascular diseases loom larger, and mental disorders smaller, than the averages for all nursing homes.

Marketing: Demand for nursing home beds far exceeds supply, and most experts expect the gap to remain or widen for the foreseeable future. The Administration on Aging estimates between 1990 and 2020 an additional 900,000 nursing home beds will be needed. Keeping up with this demand would require building a 123-bed nursing home facility every day during the 30-year period 1990 to 2020. The heaviest demand is projected for California, Florida, New York, Ohio, and Pennsylvania.

Occupancy rates, currently about 92 percent, have fallen somewhat lately due to soaring private-pay rates, bad publicity about nursing homes, and the increasing availability of alternative forms of care. However, the burgeoning over-75 population, as well as changes in treatment patterns encouraged by prospective payment, will continue to increase demand for skilled nursing services. Also, in states that have withdrawn certificate of need requirements, entry into the market has become easier and the number of beds has increased, driving down occupancy rates.

With this high level of demand, acquiring skilled nursing capabilities often is more problematic than filling the beds. However, many areas do feel competitive pressures, particularly in attracting the more lucrative private-pay market. Hospital discharge planners and social workers are the primary referral sources for patients entering the nursing home directly from a hospital, which is the entry point for between a third and half of all nursing home residents. These referrers can be contacted directly through phone calls and invitations to visit the nursing facility. As nursing home placement continues to become more difficult, decision-making authority is likely to rise to higher levels within the hospital, and will often include priority placement or lease arrangements.

Physicians will suggest that a patient seek skilled nursing care, but generally will not recommend a specific facility. However, a critical issue in the selection of a facility is the attending physician's willingness to travel to the home to visit the patient. Most physicians are unwilling to travel more than 15 or 20 minutes to see a patient in a nursing home, and hence the best location for a skilled nursing facility is within a short drive of the hospital.

About three-fifths of nursing home residents are admitted by their children or other relatives excluding the spouse, and nearly one-fourth are admitted from a relative's residence. Thus children and other close relatives often are the primary decision-making unit in selecting a particular nursing home. The factors that typically influence their decision include the physician's willingness to visit, the distance between the facility and their home, the financial situation of the patient and family, and the perceived quality and comfort of available care and services.

To maximize revenue, a new skilled nursing facility should be located in an area that has a relatively low ratio of SNF beds to older residents. The national average is about 57 beds per 1000 residents over 65, but this figure varies broadly by state. The national low is in Arizona with 17 certified beds per 1000 elderly, while the national high is in Minnesota, with 89 certified beds per 1000. Some experts recommend that skilled nursing bed capacity in an area should not exceed 3 to 4 percent of the over-65 population. Checking with hospital discharge planners about numbers of discharges to SNFs and their medical needs and financial resources, as well as waitlists for facilities, will provide essential information for estimating demand.

Revenue can also be enhanced by locating a facility in a community with a high proportion of potential private payers. However, this may or may not be the population that the sponsoring hospital hopes to serve. In any case, the facility must be close enough to the affiliated hospital for attending physicians to see patients conveniently.

Competition: Hospital-based skilled nursing facilities compete with SNFs associated with other hospitals, as well as with freestanding facilities. Most freestanding SNFs are proprietary, and many are owned by national chains. Less than one-tenth of hospital-owned SNFs are proprietary.

Hospital-based skilled nursing facilities have an advantage over their freestanding competitors in three respects. First, Medicare reimbursement limits are far more generous to the former. However, since Medicare usually pays for a relatively small proportion of total revenues, this advantage may be mitigated by the excess overhead carried by many hospital-based SNFs. A recent HCFA study found that although case mix intensity and staffing patterns were more costly for hospital-based than freestanding facilities, those differences accounted for only half of the cost differential; overhead allocation apparently accounts for the remainder. A second advantage for hospital-based skilled nursing facilities is their control over the referral system. Since a significant proportion of SNF patients are discharged directly from hospitals, a nearby hospital-based SNF probably will receive nearly all referrals coming from the affiliated institution. Finally, a skilled nursing facility associated with a hospital can enjoy the benefits of the hospital's reputation, an important advantage given the public's negative view—often justified—about the quality of nursing home care.

Private investors with aggressive strategies and (often) advantages of scale are capturing an increasing share of the nursing home market, primarily through purchase of existing facilities. Beverly Enterprises of Pasadena, California, the nation's largest nursing home corporation, has 1032 nursing homes with more than 113,000 beds. After years of growth, the company began selling homes in 1987. By 1988, Beverly had sold about 100 homes. In recent years, the large chains have faced declining profits because of increased labor costs, insufficient Medicaid reimbursement, and greater competition for patients.

Overall, industry competition is increasing, putting pressure on private-pay prices. Yet competition in this market is very much a local phenomenon, given the relatively small market area for skilled (as opposed to custodial) care. Many hospitals have been able to use their unique role in the referral system as a competitive advantage in the skilled nursing business.

Timetable: The feasibility analysis and market plan for a skilled nursing facility can take from several months to a year, depending on the speed at which the sponsoring organization can move. The CON approval required in most states for construction may be applied for and granted within that time frame, or may take somewhat longer; in many states, CONs are not issued at all. Once ground is broken, a typical facility (100 to 125 beds) can be completed in 15 to 18 months. Hospital-based skilled nursing facilities typically require six months to two years to develop from start to finish, with the speed of decision-making within the hospital administration being the primary determining factor.

Management: Although managing a nursing home appears to be similar to managing an acute care hospital, the resemblance can be deceiving. Staffing levels are lower, and training must emphasize sensitivity to elderly needs and restoration of function. Patients tend to be older and more physically and mentally frail. Reimbursement comes largely from Medicaid and private-pay sources rather than Medicare. Architectural design of the facility must accommodate the physical, cognitive, and perceptual needs of the elderly. These and other factors all differ from those of an acute inpatient setting. Most experts agree that the best manager of a skilled nursing facility is a person with specific experience in the long-term care industry.

For similar reasons, converting acute care beds to long-term beds—an appealing concept in a time of declining hospital census and rising nursing home occupancy—can be a difficult process to manage successfully. Economic efficiency dictates that a SNF should have about 50 patients per nursing station (many states set the limit at 60); typical hospital inpatient units have half that ratio. Also, skilled nursing care requires a less intensive level of care. Many nurses accustomed to hospital work are uncomfortable providing the lower level of care involved with skilled nursing. Finally, skilled care staff usually are paid less than inpatient staff, which can create problems when seemingly similar care is being delivered within the same building by differently paid providers.

Building, buying, or joint-venturing to acquire skilled nursing capabilities may all be reasonable courses of action, depending on individual circumstances. Purchasing or joint-venturing with an existing facility eliminates the need for CON approval, which is difficult or impossible to get in most states. These options also enable the hospital to gain needed expertise. If the nursing home is near the hospital, which it should be, the hospital may have significant bargaining power due to its status as a feeder. The hospital's threat of building a competing nursing home may also provide bargaining leverage. On the other hand, building a new home may be cheaper (depending on the area) and is more likely to result in a facility designed in accordance with hospital philosophy and current market needs.

Development Concerns: Three key elements to consider in developing a nursing home are local demographics, state regulations, and Medicaid reimbursement. A local survey should examine current and future numbers of elderly persons—particularly those over age 75—within the primary market area in relation to the number of available skilled nursing beds. Income levels for the over-65 population should also be investigated to determine the potential for a private-pay market. The supply-demand balance can easily be assessed by speaking to discharge planners and examining occupancy levels and waitlists for local nursing homes.

State certificate-of-need regulations are available from state health planning offices or local health systems agencies (HSAs). The CON laws usually require approval for capital expenditures of $750,000 or more for any nursing home construction. Many states use CON laws to restrict nursing home development despite the demand for skilled care beds; politically it is more palatable to deny applications for new construction than to reduce or contain reimbursement dollars per recipient. About 90 percent of the states currently are using regulatory mechanisms to restrict nursing home construction, including:

- temporary or permanent delays in CON approval;

- denials, which do not affect building directly, but disallow Medicare or Medicaid reimbursement for capital costs;

- refusing Medicaid reimbursement for new nursing home beds; or

- blanket moratoria on new nursing home construction.

There is a trend among some states to deregulate nursing home supply. Since 1983, 11 states have repealed their CON requirements for nursing homes. The repeal of CONs has increased competition.

For example, Arizona repealed its CON law governing nursing home construction in 1985 and experienced an explosion in new construction. Other states that have repealed CON laws for nursing homes are: Arizona, California, Colorado, Idaho, Kansas, Minnesota, New Mexico, South Dakota, Utah, and Wyoming. Louisiana never had a CON law. Although Arkansas repealed its CON law in 1987, the state established a commission that reviews building plans much like the CON review. In Montana and Ohio, the state legislatures will review their CON requirements in 1989.

Other regulatory considerations involve quality of care issues. A recently published congressional report alleged that over a third of the nation's nursing facilities are substandard. A survey by the nursing home industry itself found that as many as half of all nursing homes have been cited for violating state requirements in 1987 and 1988. The American Health Care Association, which conducted the survey, said the violations were linked to inadequate Medicaid reimbursement.

In 1987, Congress approved more rigorous inspections and harsher penalties for facilities violating nursing home standard requirements. The federal government and states must implement the new law by 1991. Pending regulations should be watched carefully to assess impact on administrative flexibility and care costs.

In addition, the HCFA has released a consumer's guide to certified nursing homes that includes information on the staff-to-patient ratios and histories of the facilities' sanctions and compliance with standards.

State legislatures are acting to improve the situation. In the first eight months of 1987, 12 states enacted legislation to protect nursing home residents' rights to improve access for Medicaid beneficiaries or increase Medicaid agencies' ability to crack down on substandard nursing homes.

State Medicaid reimbursement levels and methods are critical to the financial viability of a nursing home. SNF reimbursement rates per patient-day vary from about $30 to $150, but average around $50. The ICF reimbursement rates per patient-day vary from $28 to $150, but average around $40. State Medicaid offices can explain the reimbursement formula, wage index, and other adjustments. Some states pay prospectively, others retrospectively; some set facility-specific rates, while others use uniform class rates. States also vary in what they consider skilled care. Generally, severity of illness is not taken into consideration, although this may be included in future rate formulas as nursing homes admit increasing numbers of sicker patients. As required by the 1987 nursing home reform law, state Medicaid plans must review their nursing home rates by September 1990 to take into account the cost of implementing the new law.

Information Sources: Industry associations can provide a wealth of information on skilled nursing homes. The largest of these are The American Health Care Association, 1201 L St., N.W., Washington, DC 20005, (202) 842-4444; The American Association of Homes for the Aged, 1129 20th Street, N.W., Suite 400, Washington, DC 20036, (202) 296-5960; and The American College of Health Care Administrators, 325 South Patrick Street, Alexandria, VA 22314, (703) 549-5822.

The American Hospital Association's Section for Aging and Long-Term Care Services is knowledgeable about skilled nursing care. The address and phone number are 840 North Lake Shore Drive, Chicago, IL 60611; (312) 280-6372.

Transportation Services

Many older persons cannot or do not drive. The frail elderly who are most in need of hospital services are also the most likely to be unable to drive or to take advantage of public transportation. Many older adults live alone and far from any relatives who could drive them to medical care. For these reasons, transportation is an important adjunct to most eldercare services.

Most communities offer some form of local transportation services for older persons, often through an area agency on aging, the Red Cross, or a community action organization. Recently, an increasing number of hospitals have begun to provide transportation to patients entering or leaving their facility, and they often include on their routes nearby offices of their affiliated physicians. These services typically pick up patients who have scheduled appointments at the hospital; they are not used for emergencies. Most programs require advanced notice of 24 hours or more, but some will pick up passengers on short notice. At Mount Sinai Medical Center in Miami Beach, Florida, scheduling is handled through physician offices or hospital departments. After the doctor or department schedules the ride, the transportation department calls the patient to confirm the appointment.

Transportation programs range in size and scope. Some services have just one passenger car or only use the cars of their volunteer drivers. These programs usually transport about 25 to 30 passengers each week. At the other end of the spectrum is the Mount Sinai program, which has 15 vans and one 25-seat minibus. That program averages 320 passengers each day. The geographic area for pickup and return usually is limited to the service area of the sponsoring hospital, although some programs will transport patients outside of that area. Destinations may be limited to the hospital itself, may include medical staff offices, or may be virtually unlimited.

Most transportation programs operate on weekdays during normal business hours, when the majority of scheduled procedures take place. Volume ranges from several passengers a day to nearly 1000 per week. Most programs are free, and those that are not usually charge only nominal fees. Mount Sinai did a careful analysis of all cost factors, and came to the conclusion that, due to increases in insurance, inspections, driver training, and paperwork, it would actually cost more to collect fees than to run the service for free.

Value: Transportation services can be tremendously valuable to older adults who lack the means to travel to or from medical appointments. A substantial proportion of the frail elderly are in this situation: a 1980 study at Middlesex Memorial Hospital in Middletown, Connecticut, found that 45 percent of all persons over the age of 60 admitted for care were unable to drive. Many of those elderly were wheelchair-bound or otherwise too disabled to take advantage of public transportation. Thus, a hospital-sponsored transportation program can be quite beneficial for older persons.

Hospitals offering transportation services believe that their benefits go beyond community service, as important as that may be. They feel strongly that by facilitating the trip, transportation programs attract patients who might not otherwise use their hospital. Thus, the programs pay for themselves many times over through increased admissions. In addition, the vehicles used for transport can generate publicity and goodwill by displaying the hospital name and logo. Finally, by offering rides to and from the offices of affiliated physicians, a transportation program can promote positive relations between hospital and medical staff.

Cost: Capital costs for transportation services depend largely on vehicle costs and vary along two dimensions: program size and method of acquiring vehicles. A large 4-door sedan or station wagon might cost $10,000, a 15-passenger van $20,000, and a 25-seat minibus $50,000. However, many programs receive donations of one or more vehicles. A foundation, corporation, or local merchant—such as a bank—may subsidize the purchase of a vehicle; this can be encouraged by offering to display the organization's name on the vehicle. Auto dealerships may donate cars or vans as charitable contributions.

Operating costs can be extremely low for a transportation program. Vehicle costs average about $4 to $6 per round trip for gas, oil, maintenance, insurance, and registration, depending on the type of vehicle and the length of the average trip. Some programs estimate vehicle costs at $1.50 to $2.50 per mile. Labor is the other major expense. Smaller programs may use only volunteer drivers, but most transportation services pay their drivers, at least on a part-time basis. Compensation may be from $5 to $10 per hour, or perhaps $10,000 to $15,000 per year. Generally speaking, other overhead typically is absorbed by the hospital. Liability insurance usually is covered under the hospital policy.

Staffing: Besides some sort of coordinator, the only staff necessary for a transportation program are drivers. Some or all of these may volunteer their services. One small (two-vehicle) program in California has just six volunteers. Drivers might not have any qualifications other than a driver's license. Established programs often require a chauffeur's license and train their drivers in first aid and other skills. Because drivers often assist passengers in moving in and out of the vehicle and to and from the door of the destination, and sometimes even around the hospital, it is ideal to have drivers who are physically sturdy. The eight drivers for Mount Sinai's program handle most intrahospital transports, thus, greatly reducing the need to hire aides to move patients to and from units. In fact,

Mount Sinai's paid, uniformed drivers all start inside the hospital, then move up to working outside. This makes them fairly knowledgeable about the hospital's operations. They can answer patients' questions and act as representatives of the hospital.

Larger programs hire a dispatcher to schedule trips and keep track of vehicles. An administrator and some secretarial or clerical support is needed, but the time required may be so minimal for smaller programs that these responsibilities can be added to existing positions. In many hospitals, the auxiliary sponsors and manages the transportation program.

Revenues: Most transportation programs do not charge for their services and generate no revenues whatsoever. Some programs ask for nominal donations, usually from $1.00 to $3.00, but this will not raise more than a few thousand dollars annually at most. A few transportation services charge fees, usually averaging about $5 a ride. This practice may generate revenues of $10,000 to $40,000 annually, a sum that is unlikely to add up to more than half the costs of operating the vehicles. For instance, at El Camino Hospital in Mountain View, California, riders are charged from a minimum of $3 to a maximum of $8, depending upon the distance. Riders needing the handicap lift van are charged $20 to $30. The volunteer driver gives the rider an envelope with the amount written on it, to mail payment to the office. Reminder statements are sent out at the end of each month. Most program managers feel that the revenues gained from increased use of hospital services outweighs money lost on operating costs, and they do not care to risk the loss of an admission for a few dollars.

Market: Primary users of transportation services are the frail elderly living alone, who do not drive. Not all passengers are elderly or frail, but those characteristics increase the likelihood that an individual would need the service. Smaller transportation programs emphasize scheduled inpatient visits to the sponsoring hospital and, therefore, tend to serve many patients needing dialysis, radiation therapy, and physical therapy.

Although most programs focus on users of hospital and medical services, some cast their nets more widely. Mount Sinai Medical Center started its transportation program to pick up volunteers to encourage them to donate their services. Although most of its current passengers are patients, volunteers remain welcome to use the service.

Marketing: Currently, few hospital-based transportation programs are heavily promoted. In existing promotional programs, three techniques predominate. First, the name of the sponsoring hospital typically is displayed prominently on all vehicles. Second, promotional posters and brochures are placed around the hospital and the community, and announcements are made in inhouse hospital publications. Third, the medical staff is contacted so that they will encourage patients to use the service. This may involve a simple open house and promotional placards placed in physician offices.

Local area agencies on aging should be familiar with a hospital's transportation program, since they often sponsor information and referral publications or taped phone messages. Members of senior organizations can be made aware of available services through newsletters or announcements. The adult children of frail elderly can be notified of the program through caregiver support groups and corporate inhouse newsletters.

Competition: Transportation for older adults is not a competitive business, particularly when the route is to and from a hospital. Although the alternatives to a hospital-based transportation program include driving oneself, using public transit, or calling a taxi, the first is impossible for many older persons, the second is impractical, and the third is more expensive than a hospital service. Other possibilities involve transportation services offered by AAAs and community organizations. The only competition that a hospital might be concerned with would be a similar transportation program at another hospital, which conceivably could motivate some patient to use the services of the competing institution. In the Miami Beach area, three other hospitals have recently added transportation services in order to "keep up with" Mount Sinai.

Timetable: A transportation program can be established fairly quickly. A vehicle can be acquired and a driver hired within a few weeks, and service can start immediately thereafter. However, the availability of transportation services does not translate into demand for those services until potential passengers become aware of the program. Therefore, the critical issue in regard to time is marketing. A transportation program should be premarketed to physicians, discharge planners, elder representatives, and hospital staff before and immediately after service becomes available so as to encourage utilization from the start.

Management: Most transportation programs require relatively little management time or expertise. Few hospitals have any individual truly managing their program: often a secretary or volunteer contacts drivers when rides are requested. Larger programs use dispatchers to monitor van locations and service requests. Frequently, responsibility for the program rests with the auxiliary, which often sponsors and subsidizes the service.

Development Concerns: Insurance for drivers and vehicles is an important concern in operating a transportation program. While insurance regulations vary by state, it is essential that the program as a whole be covered so that the financial burden of an accident does not fall on the driver or the hospital. This is especially important to consider when volunteers drive the vehicles. At El Camino Hospital in Mountain View, California, management of the Road Runners transportation service was recently shifted from the auxiliary to the hospital for insurance purposes.

A large proportion of passengers will be frail, and some will be confined to wheelchairs. Therefore it is ideal to have at least one vehicle, probably a van, that has a wheelchair lift. This adds perhaps a thousand dollars to the cost of the van, but is safer than lifting a person into the vehicle and saves a great deal of driver time and energy.

Information Sources: Local area agencies on aging are the best sources of information about available transportation services for elders. Community organizations that sponsor programs can provide details about challenges and opportunities of the local market, although some may view hospitals as competitors.

Hospitals considering establishing a major transportation program should contact the Manager of Transportation at Mount Sinai Medical Center, 4300 Alton Road, Miami Beach, FL 33140; (305) 674-2535.

Valet Parking

For some older persons at some hospitals, walking from the parking lot to the main entry can be difficult or exhausting. Although most hospitals allow visitors to be dropped off at the front door, this is not sufficient for the older adult driving himself or herself or for the frail elderly couple. In addition, parking spaces may be in short supply or somewhat distant from the building entrance. Due to these and other reasons, some hospitals—especially those with restricted parking or large lots—offer valet parking service.

Valet services take two forms. The traditional system is similar to that of some restaurants: the car is driven to the front door, the attendant takes the key, gives the driver a numbered token and parks the car. At the conclusion of the hospital visit, the driver gives the token to the attendant, who then retrieves the car. San Jose Health Center in San Jose, California, has such a service. A different system is similar to that of some amusement parks: drivers park their own cars and are picked up by a golf cart or tram, which shuttles them to and from the hospital entry as needed. Examples of this type of service can be found at Walter O. Boswell Memorial Hospital in Sun City, Arizona, and at Palomar Hospital in Escondido, California.

Either system is inexpensive to establish and operate, and can be staffed partly or entirely by volunteers. Although the latter system requires the acquisition of a vehicle, golf carts are much less expensive than cars or vans, and purchase often can be subsidized by donations. Valet parking services offer a significant convenience to patients and visitors. By making the hospital more accessible, the service also encourages utilization and promotes an image of caring for and reaching out to older adults and others.

Eldercare Case Studies

4

The rapidly changing demographic landscape has left many health care providers scrambling for models on which to base the development of eldercare services. Fortunately, several far-sighted health care organizations anticipated the age wave and have established leading eldercare programs that address the needs of older adults creatively and effectively. This section examines six of them.

None of these programs claim to be perfect, nor do they claim to have fully matured. However, all have been highly successful in navigating uncharted eldercare waters through turbulent demographic seas in today's stormy health care climate. This section provides a detailed view of how several organizations have approached the challenges of eldercare in their communities and what results they have seen to date.

CASE STUDY 1
Baptist Medical Center's Third Age Life Center

Comprehensive Senior Program
Aims at Fuller Life

The former president of Oklahoma City's nonprofit, 577-bed Baptist Medical Center, Philip A. Newbold, felt that his institution needed to respond to a distinct demographic challenge: the population was getting older. Newbold and his staff recognized that the burgeoning older adult market will have a dramatic financial impact on America's health care providers. After serious research and brainstorming, they created the Third Age Life Center to provide a comprehensive set of services geared to older adults.

Research began in February 1986, with hospital staff, physicians, and community representatives meeting to repackage existing services and create new ones. After more than 2000 man-hours, involving the talents of 200 people, the Third Age Life Center opened in October 1986, offering 22 of the 36 services the research had originally identified.

The term "third age" refers to the concept that life has three stages: first age (birth to 24), a period of survival and growth; second age (25 to 65), a period of work and production; and third age (65 +), a period of expanded enjoyment, companionship, purpose, and fulfillment.

The Third Age Life Center links health care and life-style services to:

- create an atmosphere where older adults may reach personal fulfillment,

- create services that are both financially viable and necessary to the community, and

- provide ongoing medical research and education.

The Third Age Life Center is based on identifying services, regrouping them and, in many cases, changing the service to satisfy the Third Age Life concept: making sure the whole culture of the organization meets the unique needs of older people.

Almost every department in Baptist Medical Center is affected, since all of them have older customers. Before the center opened, about 2500 Baptist Medical Center employees went through a four-hour training program to dispel their stereotypes and myths about the elderly.

Housed in its own building, the Third Age Life Center includes the aging resource center, a community conference center, an older adult art gallery, administrative offices, and space for housing physicians specializing in care for older adults and, possibly, community agencies who might want to move in.

Membership Program: The key component of the center, and the entry point for all of its other services, is a free membership program, LIFEPASS, which covers everything from health care and finance to living arrangements and personal philosophy. Within the first six weeks, LIFEPASS had enrolled more than 5000 members. Membership enrollment is far ahead of projections, and the program now has more than 15,000 members age 55 or older. Health and wellness activities are held on a regular basis. The ongoing enrichment series of health and life-style activities is held in a conference center, with standing-room-only attendance of 300 every month. LIFEPASS benefits include:

- savings on certain medical services, pharmacy items, durable medical equipment, breast screening, and osteoporosis screening;

- savings in local stores, a fitness center, and a gift gallery;

- a 10-percent cafeteria discount;

- free parking, and a 50-percent discount in transportation to the hospital;

- eligibility to stay in the hospital hotel for patients and their families; and

- insurance counseling, and assistance in filing claims.

The opening of the Baptist program included public announcements, a press conference, and seminar by Ken Dychtwald, Ph.D., on the aging of America. Television, radio, and newspaper announcements were used for six weeks, during which time 5000 members were signed up. Since the opening, no media time has been purchased, and primary marketing methods have been by word-of-mouth and through physicians and community agencies.

The strongest referral source right now is members' word of mouth; followed second by the admissions office, where the clerk provides eligible patients with LIFEPASS applications during the admission; and third, by the hospital's physicians. Applications continue to pour in at the rate of 100 to 125 per week.

The LIFEPASS program has three full-time employees, plus college interns and volunteers, who were immediately interested in helping with the program.

Staffing: The Third Age Life Center staff includes the director, who reports to the operational vice president, an assistant director, an outreach services coordinator, two LIFEPASS advisers, a care coordinator, and an administrative assistant. The resource center and library are staffed by volunteers.

Advisory Board: A national advisory board consisting of well-known experts on aging, including Christiaan Barnard, M.D., Ken Dychtwald, Ph.D., and pollster George Gallup, Jr., was formed to consult on the center's development. That voluntary group meets on an annual basis, and is available informally for advice.

Packaging Services: The whole Third Age Life Center program has been so successful that in August 1987, Baptist created a new division of marketing, Third Age Life National Marketing Services, to carry the concept to other institutions.

National Marketing Services' mandate is to offer hospitals six essential services packaged as instructional manuals for creating a comprehensive older adult program. The marketing arm was formed to generate revenues, which will go back into developing new programs for the Third Age Life Center. New programs will also be repackaged and made available to other hospitals.

The six essential services are the:

1. *planning model,* for developing an older adult program of services tailored to each community;

2. *market research model,* to assist in collecting and understanding useful data;

3. *sensitivity training manual,* to dispel myths and change stereotypical attitudes employees may have about older people;

4. *care coordination program,* to coordinate needed services so that older people can remain as independent as possible, as long as possible;

5. *LIFEPASS enrollment program*, to meet both the health care and life-style needs of older adults and serve as their central information resource; and the

6. *marketing communication manual*, which details how this growing market segment responds to various media, programs, and messages.

Housed in a building next to the Third Age Life Center, the marketing department has three full-time employees and plans to use volunteers in a telemarketing role. Third Age Life National Marketing Services currently has program components being developed or put to use in Oklahoma, Kentucky, New Jersey, and Indiana.

Information Source: Lucinda McMullen, Assistant Director, Third Age Life Center, Baptist Medical Center of Oklahoma, 3300 Northwest Expressway, Oklahoma City, OK 73112-4481; (405) 946-9235.

CASE STUDY 2
Baylor Health Care System's Baylor 55Plus^R

Telemarketing Database
Supports Membership Program Success

When Al Swinney says that Baylor Health Care System's senior membership program has generated $23,225,778 in new patient revenue during its first year of operation, he is not making a seat-of-the-pants estimate. Swinney is Baylor's senior vice president for marketing and strategic management.

At the core of Baylor's exceptionally successful senior membership program (and of its other programs as well) is its telemarketing system, a minicomputer with 40 dumb terminals that can, said Swinney, "capture an unlimited amount of information." Each product has a set of screens that display demographic, media, and other data for its particular database.

Using this system, the membership program, 55Plus, has built a user database that permits it to break down its membership in terms of gender, insurance coverage, age, and other specific categories. This database not only generates a list of people to whom other Baylor health care products and services can be marketed, it also allows the program to offer its members more efficient service. When members call in with a question, the necessary information can immediately be accessed; callers can be told precisely where and how to get what they want based on their location and other needs.

Efficient Tracking: This system enables 55Plus to track the cost-effectiveness of promotional efforts in different media, the utilization rate of various services, and the user rate generated for other Baylor services. And when it comes down to cost/benefit to the Baylor system, this program has more than anecdotes to offer. It has the figures.

When Baylor started its senior membership program in January 1987, its goal was 8000 members in the first year—44,176 signed up. During that same year, 8982 hospital admissions were generated from this membership, 31.2 percent of whom were not former Baylor patients.

The program has been implemented in all seven of the Baylor system's hospitals in north Texas. The proportion of those over 65 in this total service area is 9 percent. Forty percent of its patient volume (in days) represents persons over 65.

The idea behind 55Plus was to create a program to begin to tie people into the facility at the beginning of their high-demand years. The program was conceived as part of Baylor's overall goal of relating to its customers in terms of their extended value over a health care lifetime.

Inpatient Benefits: Benefits for members who are hospitalized include: visits from guest representatives who answer questions on hospital policies or financial assistance and resolve problems that arise during hospitalization; transportation to and from the hospital; free parking, TV, and telephone service; private room accommodations at semiprivate room rates; complimentary guest meals for a visiting family member or friend; and interest-free payment plans to finance the balance of hospital bills after insurance coverage.

Other Benefits: Benefits for nonhospitalized members include: assistance with insurance filing; physician referral service (20 to 30 percent of members entered the program without a personal physician—1880 members were referred during the first year); complimentary home health care visits (up to six hours) for homemaker services after discharge; free or discounted health screenings and health seminars held at a variety of locations in the service area; a quarterly newsletter; and discounts on health-related goods and services such as prescription eyewear.

Figures from the program's first year of operation show that the most highly used benefits tend to be those that are tangible and simple like free parking (used 81,244 times) and guest meals (used 44,071 times). Swinney said that benefits with high-level perceptual value bring in members even when these benefits are not highly utilized. Only 114 members, for example, were transported to and 494 from the hospital; and payment plans were utilized by only 141 members. The discounted private room also has a high perceptual value (members took advantage of this discount for 47,919 days), but this benefit costs the hospital relatively little. Swinney said the difference is only $8 or $9 more per day and that most rooms are private anyway.

Promotion: The program was launched with 30-second television ads featuring specific benefits, followed immediately by double-page, highly detailed newspaper ads. Later, direct mail was used to penetrate particular zip codes. Television ads are now used only occasionally to keep the program in the public's awareness.

Response to advertising is routinely tracked on a week-by-week basis and modifications are made accordingly. If a newspaper ad is not getting a certain minimal level of response, for instance, it will be pulled even if the plan was to run it for several weeks. Direct mail has been most efficient in driving a response—a call in for a booklet or application. Total advertising expenditures were $60,000 at the start of the program in January 1987, but had dropped to $5000 by the end of the year.

Press releases are sent to newspapers, television stations, radio news programs, senior agencies, and area churches, and presentations are given at local AARP chapters, church groups, and various senior organizations.

Its program director is the only full-time employee of 55Plus. The 12 full-time employees who operate the telemarketing system service all other Baylor programs as well. Swinney says that when Baylor's planners conceived this membership program, they "deliberately didn't want to create another layer. The idea was to get more out of what we already do—to integrate this program with existing departments." He considers it essential for any hospital considering a membership program to have a telemarketing system in place: "The value of a membership program is in that database."

Baylor is selling its senior membership program (not including the computer system) to other hospitals for $35,000; it also sells the telemarketing system (hardware, software, and support) customized to the buyer's needs.

Information Source: Vice President, Resource Sales or Director of Contract Sales, Baylor Health Care System, 3201 Worth Street, Dallas, TX 75226; (800) 999-5460 or (214) 820-2895.

CASE STUDY 3
Walter O. Boswell Memorial Hospital's Volunteers

Volunteers Perform Roles
Inside and Outside Hospital

Soon after a *Fortune*-500 company senior vice president stepped down, he began another career, preparing videotapes for the employees of Walter O. Boswell Community Hospital in Sun City, Arizona—as a volunteer.

This talented, high-powered man brought his volunteer services to the right place. At Boswell, volunteers are taken very seriously, and are assigned jobs based upon their skills and interests. With 2200 volunteers—1500 of those active on a weekly basis—Boswell runs the largest hospital volunteer organization in Arizona. Fewer than 10 percent of its volunteers dropped away in 1987. Among those who left, sickness or death ranked as the top causes.

Variety of Tasks: A retired engineer helps insure that hazardous materials are properly stored; a former teacher reviews training manuals. Other volunteers drive courtesy carts from the parking lot so patients and visitors will not have to climb the hill on hot summer days. Standing near the front door, volunteers greet guests. Upstairs, in a patient's room, volunteers help write letters for patients or serve coffee and danish. Other volunteers carry drugs from the pharmacy to the nurses, wards, units, and nurse's station.

More than 100 tasks are performed by volunteers. In 1987, their hours tallied 250,000. Since the hospital was formed 20 years ago, volunteers have given three million hours. On any given day, volunteers usually outnumber staff, although they never give out medications or administer patient care.

Outside the Hospital: Outside Boswell's walls, volunteers perform other kinds of work for the hospital in this affluent retirement community. Besides manning the senior center and library, they take blood pressure readings at health fairs, share information with newly diagnosed cancer patients and their families, and work at arts and crafts shops in nearby shopping centers. Recently the 355-bed hospital opened an aging resource center, which is manned with volunteers.

Acting as goodwill ambassadors, Boswell's volunteers greet new residents of Sun City, sharing information about the hospital, senior center, and long-term care facility. Their goal is to make newcomers understand that the medical complex belongs to them.

Volunteers have become an integral part of the hospital's strategic plan. Whenever the hospital starts a new service, it searches for volunteers to play a role in it.

Revenues: The volunteers also join the auxiliary and pay a $5 annual fee. Since its founding in 1968, the auxiliary has raised $1.8 million for hospital equipment from gift shop, thrift shop, and arts and crafts shops revenue. Auxiliary members receive a monthly newsletter and can attend classes on breast self-examination, vitamins, home blood pressure equipment, and colorectal cancer screening.

Recruitment: The hospital relies on the community to spread the word, rather than running advertisements. Articles are placed in local newspapers. Also, volunteers are encouraged to bring a friend to membership coffee klatches. Later, newcomers are interviewed, then attend a three-hour orientation. Some receive more intense training, depending upon their assignment.

Information Source: Director of Volunteer Services, Walter O. Boswell Memorial Hospital, P.O. Box 1690, 10401 Thunderbird Boulevard, Sun City, AZ 85372; (602) 876-5387.

CASE STUDY 4

East Jefferson General Hospital's Elder Advantage

Membership Program
Based on Market Research

In 1985, East Jefferson General Hospital, a 557-bed nonprofit community hospital, found itself in an unfamiliar—and uncomfortable—position. Until then, it had dominated its local market, New Orleans's major suburban community. But in 1985, two for-profit hospitals opened in East Jefferson's service area, and, in 1987, a third for-profit joined the competition.

In an attempt to preserve its market share, the hospital conducted careful market research, which showed that its 130,000-household, middle- and upper middle-class, residential service area was aging. The only growth was among the over-50 population.

The research identified three distinct target populations:

1. the financially secure, healthy, and independent elderly who made up 60 to 70 percent of the total senior population;

2. the frail, homebound elders afflicted with chronic illnesses who accounted for 20 to 30 percent; and

3. the adult children of the frail elderly—the caregivers.

To capture this market and retain the loyalty of its physicians, the hospital decided to develop a membership program for the elderly. Currently, East Jefferson offers a skilled nursing facility, a home care program, and a geriatric psychiatric program, and it plans to add other services for the elderly in the future.

Information from focus groups of seniors was used to determine the scope and benefits of the program. Even the name, Elder Advantage, grew out of these sessions: participants responded positively to "elder," with its associations with elder statesman or church elder. Focus groups are a continuing part of the marketing effort, providing feedback that is used to refine the program.

The program started in the fall of 1986 with the goal of signing up 5000 members in the first year. More than 7300 joined. As of

September 1988, membership had exceeded 13,000 and was growing at a rate of about 100 per week.

Benefits: The program's core benefits, and the ones Jamie Haeuser, the hospital's administrative associate for marketing, says are the biggest draws are: no bill for inpatient services if the patient carries Medicare A and B and supplemental insurance, and professional assistance with filing for insurance. Other benefits include:

- four free health screenings annually (for glaucoma, diabetes, foot problems, and colon cancer);

- free blood pressure screenings;

- free private room upgrade;

- discounts on low sodium, low fat, calorie-controlled frozen meals;

- community education classes;

- Care Ring Service, a once-a-day phone call to members who live alone and cannot get out;

- a daily visit to hospitalized members from the program coordinator who helps the patient negotiate the system; and

- community resource referrals.

Promotion: The initial promotion of Elder Advantage was to solicit inquiries and establish name recognition. This was done through newspaper and radio ads that attempted to convey the tangible benefits of the program to potential members. Late-night and early-morning radio spots were found to be a very good way to reach seniors, who often suffer from insomnia and listen to the radio during these times. Costs for advertising and direct-mail promotion, which run an estimated $15 per member, are covered by membership fees.

The program coordinator has spoken about the program to diverse groups of elders, taking advantage of the fact that seniors tend to belong to organizations and groups. Haeuser says "a lot of attention" was given to the program brochure, which was placed in doctors' offices and in public places around the hospital, and mailed to outside locations such as bingo halls. Additionally, admitting department personnel were enlisted to alert seniors to the program and its benefits.

AARP Chapter: The hospital worked with the local chapter of the AARP from the beginning, and has now formed two chapters of its own, with some 250 members in each.

Direct Mail and Telemarketing: The core of the recruitment campaign is the use of direct mail in conjunction with telemarketing. Two direct-mail pieces are sent to the target population, then followed up by calls from volunteers—themselves elderly—who ask whether the person has received the mailers and if he or she has any questions.

This technique, according to Haeuser, has outpulled straight advertising three-to-one in bringing in new members. Because of the personal touch it adds, Haeuser considers it a definite advantage to use elderly volunteers rather than professional telemarketers. The team of about 20 volunteers worked with the coordinator to develop the system; they are trained by the coordinator or by each other. The same volunteers also help with enrollment and mailing.

Membership Fee: Although Elder Advantage is competing with four other elder membership programs in the New Orleans area (three of which are free), the hospital has chosen to charge a membership fee of $25 per person and $30 per couple. The rationale is twofold: (1) it establishes a value-quality relationship that positions Elder Advantage as the best program available; and (2) the financial tie with the hospital is a way to ensure that members will choose East Jefferson for admission when they have a choice. Because they have an investment in the hospital, it matters where they go—and they know they will get the inpatient benefits.

Physician Involvement: The program has an advisory group consisting of physicians with large numbers of elderly patients. Doctors are frequently updated and asked for their input on each aspect of the program. Many physicians have received referrals of new patients as a result of the program, since 30 percent of new members do not have a personal physician. (Many have outlived their doctors and have not had a health problem serious enough to require them to find a new one.)

All doctors of new members, even those not affiliated with the hospital, receive postcards informing them that their patients have joined Elder Advantage. Hospital-affiliated physicians also are given certificates to place in their offices stating that they are participants in the program.

Staffing: Elder Advantage employed two full-time staff during its first year, and has now added a third. The coordinator, herself an elder, is a nurse with senior management experience. She keeps hospital executives apprised of what is current in the field of geriatrics so this information can be used in future strategic planning. The insurance/billing specialist has 20 years experience in Medicare. The third full-time employee helps with the insurance program. Haeuser believes that having a professional insurance counselor significantly enhances the quality of the program and is one of the features that gives Elder Advantage its competitive edge.

Revenues: Jamie Haeuser estimates that the program has generated $13 million in patient revenue for the hospital. This estimate is based on the number of members who have been hospitalized and takes into account the fact that half of the membership did not have existing medical record numbers. The hospital is packaging and selling this program to other hospitals for $7500. The purpose, according to Haeuser, is to build a network of hospitals offering the same basic benefits for members who travel (Elder Advantage members are frequent travelers, she says) and to expand the hospital's national networking with other institutions.

Information Source: Administrative Associate for Marketing, East Jefferson General Hospital, 4200 Houma Boulevard, Metairie, LA 70006; (504) 889-7124.

CASE STUDY 5
Huntington Hospital's Senior Care Network

Case Management Program
Invests Inherited Wealth Wisely

Almost a century ago, a vast railroad fortune helped lay the foundations for Huntington Hospital in Pasadena, California. But it was like a bolt from the blue when the 606-bed not-for-profit regional medical center discovered its name in the 1984 will of Margaret Bundy Scott. That community-minded woman had left half her $185 million estate to a group of nine local organizations, under a trust designed to enable them to fund innovative programs for children, the handicapped, and the elderly over a 10-year period.

Huntington, which had recently been turned down for a funding grant, dusted off its ambitious plan to develop a three-pronged array of geriatric services aimed at:

- health promotion and consumer education,

- case management and referrals, and

- professional education and system enhancement.

Now in its fourth year, Huntington's Senior Care Network is widely regarded as one of the best conceived, best run, and most comprehensive eldercare programs in the United States. Its original staff of four has expanded by a factor of 10, and the annual budget now tops $3 million (about $800,000 of that in 1988 was provided by the Bundy Scott Fund).

Under the rubric of health promotion and education, Huntington has established a membership program "to help people plan to be 100. Our conceptual base," said Monika White, Senior Care Network's associate director, "is to help people identify the risks of aging and age well."

Radio and Television: Effectively employing a variety of media, not least among them weekly radio and television shows, the membership program signed up over 13,500 participants within six months. Senior volunteers and a nearby junior college station produce the radio show, called *Coming of Age*, under the direction of White's staff. She estimates the cost to Senior Care Network to be about $1000 monthly. Roughly the same amount is spent on the television program, *To Your Health*, which is broadcast weekly over six Southern California cable services from Senior Care Network's own inhouse studio staffed by a full-time media specialist.

"We determined to use the money from the Bundy Scott Fund as much as possible for enduring kinds of things," said White. That's why a full-scale TV studio was outfitted and even a satellite dish installed. The latter enables the hospital to stage teleconferences for their professionals and the community. White described it as "system capacity building."

As part of the third prong in the Network program continuum—professional education and system enhancement—Senior Care Network puts on special educational programs for nurses, van drivers, homemakers and other front-line eldercare service providers.

The central element in the Senior Care Network design is the brokering of community health and social services for the elderly through a broad and sophisticated referral and case management capability. The Network serves as case manager for low-income frail elderly and disabled participants in two state-funded programs designed to keep people out of institutions. Known as the Multipurpose Senior Services Program (MSSP) and the Linkages Program, they provide Senior Care Network with $1.1 million in combined annual revenues. This covers, among other things, the cost of buying services for 200 participants in each category.

As an adjunct to these programs for qualifiers with limited financial resources (the 400 in MSSP and Linkages), the Network has added a fee-for-service case management component and, with grant funding, an ability to subsidize case management for another 100 needy applicants. Participants are directed to the proper program through a central intake system after a 20-minute telephone interview by a licensed social worker. Senior Care Network employs 16 case managers—most with master's degrees in social work or RN degrees—who carefully ascertain clients' needs before linking them with providers.

"We don't believe in just giving out phone numbers," said White, "and we don't think most people even ask the right questions when they call. People tend to spend too much or not enough on care. Our philosophy is that the elderly need to preserve their energy, their strength and their assets."

Fees: About 75 clients make use of the fee-for-service program at any one time, said White. Originally they were charged $125 for a home visit or $95 for an office assessment, and $60 an hour in six-minute increments for case management services. Now, however, the Network is experimenting with a number of new package rates under which participants pay a flat one-time fee of from $300 to $1000 for varying bundles of assessment, care planning, implementation, and monitoring.

Marketing: Marketing the intangible middleman services involved in case management, and holding onto clients who resent bills from an agency that cannot be seen "doing" anything, have been difficult, said White. To reach potential beneficiaries who can most readily afford it—elderly residents of exclusive estate enclaves like San Marino—White has enlisted the aid of influential Senior Care Network advisory council members in amassing a mailing list and developing materials persuasive to such an audience.

Senior Care Network has tried very hard to develop individualized marketing methods aimed at winning influential allies throughout the community. For instance, the advisory council put on the Senior Prom, a lavish socialite ball more than a year in the planning, which raised $265,000 in a single, highly publicized night. Now the council is developing plans for an endowment that will take over when the 10-year Bundy Scott grant runs out. In addition, the hospital has designated the proceeds of its fashionable thrift shop—which often acts as appraiser, consignee, and auctioneer of goods and estates in probate—as income for the Network.

Contracts with Providers: In its case management capacity, Senior Care Network has signed contracts with about one-third of the service providers in the area, said White. "We buy a lot from them, and we believe in negotiating good prices. We promised them we wouldn't compete, but would broker and coordinate their services. But it took endless open houses and luncheons and technical assistance and a quarterly newsletter to build to the present level of cooperation," White said.

While the Bundy Scott Fund has been a huge factor in the success of the ambitious Huntington program, today it is only one of a dozen funding sources. "Any amount of money will help," acknowledged White, "but you've got to use the money to leverage support."

Information Source: Associate Director, Senior Care Network, Huntington Hospital, 1837 South Fair Oaks, Pasadena, CA 91105; (818) 397-3110.

CASE STUDY 6
Senior HealthLink's OASIS

Store Center
Proves Valuable in Marketing Eldercare

On the tenth floor of the busy Meier & Frank department store in downtown Portland, Oregon, a white-haired woman stoops to squint into the viewfinder of a tripod-mounted television camera. This is not the electronics department, and she is not shopping. The woman is learning the nuts and bolts of TV program production along with a dozen or so elderly classmates at HealthLink's popular OASIS center.

OASIS—the Older Adult Service and Information System—was developed with federal funding in St. Louis in 1982 by Marylen Mann, a former teacher and community activist. She now directs a program that has expanded to more than a dozen other U.S. cities. Since 1984, OASIS has been affiliated with the Washington University School of Medicine, the Jewish Hospital of St. Louis, and the locally headquartered May Department Stores Company, one of the nation's largest retail chains.

The May Department Stores Company, indeed, was the catalyst in OASIS' growth. It has contributed both funds—more than $200,000 in 1986—and significant space in stores it owns for use as dedicated facilities for local informational, cultural, and educational services to the elderly.

Because the May Company is still expanding, there is enormous potential for the OASIS program to grow. Founder Mann expects to have established centers in 20 cities by the end of 1989.

Though OASIS' St. Louis office provides central administration and program standards supervision, each OASIS center is operated by its own community advisory committee, many of which are under the sponsorship of a local health care institution.

In Portland, OASIS is sponsored by HealthLink, a consortium of four of the area's 12 major hospitals—Emanuel Hospital and Health Center, Holladay Park Medical Center, Meridian Park Hospital, and Mount Hood Medical Center—plus an HMO; Bestcare; a preferred provider organization (PPO), CareMark; and a home care provider, the Visiting Nurse Association.

The elevator doors at Meier & Frank first opened to the comfortably furnished OASIS reception area, lounge, coordinator's office, library/information center and spacious classroom in late 1985. Since then, the Portland center has welcomed more than 22,000 elderly visitors, with an average age of 75. Among them have been 12,626 enrollees in 783 free classes ranging from acting and art to poetry reading and musical exercise. Another 10,158 of the enrollees have been participants in special events including luncheons, group birthday parties, films, lectures, and excursions.

Open from 10 AM to 3 PM Monday through Friday, the center is staffed by the equivalent of one full-time employee. Monday mornings are devoted to the training of volunteers, who provide the actual services to members. Some 3006 members have signed up at no charge. Volunteers teach all classes; by October 1988 they had donated 23,906 hours to the program.

Of several hospitals on the original advisory committee, only the HealthLink consortium was willing to assume the ongoing operational burden of the Portland OASIS. Nancy Connors, who oversees the program, said the hospitals that demurred are "very sorry now." The OASIS center, she noted, has proved a key design resource and marketing channel for Senior HealthLink, a booming $10 annual membership program launched in November 1987. (With 1,500 members signed on in the first three months, Connors hopes eventually to have a roster of 10,000.)

Costs: A typical center, according to OASIS, costs a minimum of about $25,000 to $60,000 annually to run, and the national organization charges an initial fee—usually $25,000—to coordinate the set-up of its program. HealthLink contributes some $35,000 a year to the operation of the more comprehensive OASIS center at Meier & Frank, and the national OASIS organization some $15,000. The center was established with a $50,000 seed grant from the area agency on aging. Besides the space itself, Meier & Frank contributes printing, and covers certain other expenses.

Benefits: The HealthLink program offers free health screenings, mail-order pharmacy services, eyeglasses, hearing aids, health seminars and travel, a quarterly newsletter, and free counseling on insurance, finance, home care, legal and housing matters to people over 55. In addition, Senior HealthLink offers its four member hospitals strategic planning, program development, and marketing services geared to older clients.

The affiliation of OASIS and HealthLink has been beneficial to both. OASIS has given high visibility to HealthLink programs and facilities, according to Connors. For instance, a visit to Holladay Park's lithotripter (with a free meal in the hospital cafeteria thrown in) has become a popular OASIS excursion. HealthLink staff physicians who speak at OASIS gain exposure to potential patients—and an education as they are listen to elders' probing questions in an environment quite different from an examining room.

Connors does not yet have "quantifiable data" to show the benefits to HealthLink of its expenditures on OASIS. Recently, however, she has begun to track hospital utilization by participants in Senior HealthLink and its associated activities, including OASIS.

Input from Elders: Connors has relied heavily on the focus group and test marketing input of OASIS members and volunteers in designing the program components, scope of service, and promotional and advertising materials for Senior HealthLink. (Among other things, she noted, they strongly preferred the term "seniors" to "elders," and were far more concerned with how healthy the photo models looked than their age.)

Indeed, OASIS volunteers serve as Senior HealthLink advertising models, and they staff its booths at health fairs. "They're a very effective group of people," said Connors. "Our sponsorship of OASIS has been of real direct person-to-person value. I know it has generated tremendous good will for us, too."

Information Sources: Director for Senior HealthLink, HealthLink, 500 North East Multnomah, Portland, OR 97232; (503) 239-1270, or Executive Director, Older Adult Service and Information System, 4511 Forest Park Boulevard, St. Louis, MO 63108; (314) 454-0113.

Directory of Information Sources

Associations, Organizations, and Publications

Academy of Health Services Marketing
(American Marketing Association)
250 South Wacker Drive,
  Suite 200
Chicago, IL 60606
(312) 648-0536

Alzheimer's Disease and
  Related Disorders Association
70 East Lake Street, Suite 600
Chicago, IL 60601
(312) 853-3060

American Aging Association
42nd and Dewey Avenue
Omaha, NE 68105
(402) 559-4416

American Association of Homes
  for the Aging
1129 20th Street, N.W.,
  Suite 400
Washington, DC 20036
(202) 296-5960

American Association
  of Retired Persons
1909 K Street, N.W.
Washington, DC 20049
(202) 872-4700

American Cancer Society
National Headquarters
1599 Clifton Road
Atlanta, GA 30329
(404) 320-3333

American College
  of Health Care Administrators
8120 Woodmont Avenue, Suite 200
Bethesda, MD 20814
(301) 652-8384

American Congress
  of Rehabilitation Medicine
130 South Michigan Avenue,
  Suite 1310
Chicago, IL 60603
(312) 922-9368

247

American Dental Association
211 East Chicago Avenue
Chicago, IL 60611
(312) 440-2701

American Diabetes Association, Inc.
1660 Duke Street
Alexandria, VA 22314
(703) 549-1500

American Diabetic Association
208 South LaSalle Street, Suite 1100
Chicago, IL 60604-1003
(312) 899-0040

American Foundation
for the Blind, Inc.
15 West 16th Street
New York, NY 10011
(212) 620-2000

American Geriatric Society
770 Lexington Avenue, Suite 400
New York, NY 10021
(212) 308-1414

American Health Care Association
1201 L Street
Washington, DC 20005
(202) 842-4444

American Health Foundation
320 East 43rd Street
New York, NY 10017
(212) 953-1900

American Heart Association
7320 Greenville Avenue
Dallas, TX 75231
(214) 373-6300

American Hospital Association
840 North Lake Shore Drive
Chicago, IL 60611
(312) 280-6086

American Longevity Association
243 North Lindbergh Boulevard
St. Louis, MO 63141

American Lung Association
1740 Broadway
New York, NY 10019
(212) 315-8700

American Medical Association
535 North Dearborn Street
Chicago, IL 60610
(312) 645-5000

American Occupational Therapy
Association, Inc
P.O. Box 1725
1383 Piccard Drive,
Suite 300
Rockville, MD 20850-4375
(301) 948-9626

American Pharmaceutical
Association
2215 Constitution Avenue, N.W.
Washington, DC 20037
(202) 628-4410

American Physical Therapy
Association
1111 North Fairfax Street
Alexandria, VA 22314
(703) 684-2782

American Printing House
for the Blind
P.O. Box 6085
1839 Frankfurt Avenue
Louisville, KY 40206
(502) 895-2405

American Public Health Association
1015 15th Street, N.W.
Washington, DC 20005
(202) 789-5600

American Red Cross
National Headquarters
430 17th Street, N.W.
Washington, DC 20006
(202) 737-8300

American Rheumatism Association
17 Executive Park Drive, N.E.,
  Suite 480
Atlanta, GA 30329
(404) 633-3777

American Society of Directors
  of Volunteer Services
840 North Lake Shore Drive
Chicago, IL 60611
(312) 280-6110

American Society on Aging
833 Market Street, Suite 512
San Francisco, CA 94103
(415) 543-2617

American Speech-Language-
  Hearing Association
10801 Rockville Pike
Rockville, MD 20852
(301) 897-5700

Arthritis Foundation
1314 Spring Street, N.W.
Atlanta, GA 30309
(404) 872-7100

Arthritis Information Clearinghouse
P.O. Box 9782
Arlington, VA 22209

Asociacion Nacional
  Pro Personas Mayores
Carmela G. Lacayo,
  National Executive Director
2727 West 6th Street, Suite 270
Los Angeles, CA 90057
(213) 487-1922

Asthma and Allergy Foundation
  of America
1717 Massachusetts Ave., N.W.,
  Suite 305
Washington, DC 20036
(202) 265-0265

Blue Cross and
  Blue Shield Association
676 North St. Clair
Chicago, IL 60611
(312) 440-6000

Canadian Cancer Society
77 Bloor Street, W.,
  Suite 1702
Toronto, Ontario M5S 3A1
(416) 961-7223

Canadian Cardiovascular Society
360 Victoria Avenue, Room 401
Westmount, Quebec H3Z 2N4
(514) 482-3407

Canadian Council
  of Blue Cross Plans
150 Ferrand Drive
Don Mills, Ontario M3C 1H6
(416) 429-2661

Canadian Council
  of the Blind
220 Dundas Street, Suite 610
London, Ontario N6A 1H3
(519) 433-3946

Canadian Hearing Society
271 Spadina Road
Toronto, Ontario M5R 2V3
(416) 964-9595

Canadian Heart Foundation
1 Nicholas Street, Suite 1200
Ottawa, Ontario K1N 7B7
(613) 237-4361

Canadian Hospital Association
17 York Street,
  Suite 100
Ottawa, Ontario K1N 9J6
(613) 238-8005

Canadian Lung Association
75 Albert,
  Suite 908
Ottawa, Ontario K1P 5E7
(613) 237-1208

Canadian Medical Association
P.O. Box 8650
Ottawa, Ontario K1G 0G8
(613) 731-9331

Canadian National Institute
  for the Blind
1931 Bayview Avenue
Toronto, Ontario M4G 4C8
(416) 480-7588

Canadian Pharmaceutical Association
1785 Alta Vista Drive
Ottawa, Ontario K1G 3Y6
(613) 523-7877

Canadian Public Health Association
1565 Carling Avenue,
  Suite 400
Ottawa, Ontario K1Z 8R1
(613) 725-3769

Canadian Red Cross Society
1800 Alta Vista
Ottawa, Ontario K1G 4J5
(416) 676-8000

Canadian Rehabilitation Council
  for the Disabled
1 Yonge Street,
  Suite 2110
Toronto, Ontario M5E 1E5
(416) 862-0340

Cancer Information Clearinghouse
National Cancer Institute
Office of Cancer Communications
Building 31, Room 10A-18
9000 Rockville Pike
Bethesda, MD 20892
(301) 496-5615

Catholic Health Association
  of Canada
1247 Kilbourne
Ottawa, Ontario K1H 6K9
(613) 731-7148

Catholic Health Association
  of the United States
(Formerly Catholic Hospital
  Association)
4455 Woodson Road
St. Louis, MO 63134
(314) 427-2500

Children of Aging Parents
2761 Trenton Road
Levittown, PA 19056
(215) 945-6900

Council on Education
  for Public Health
1015 15th Street, N.W.
Washington, DC 20005
(202) 789-1050

Duke University
Center for the Study of Aging
  and Human Development
Medical Center, P.O. Box 3003
Durham, NC 27710
(919) 684-8111

Eye Bank Association
  of America
1725 Eye Street, N.W., Suite 308
Washington, DC 20006
(202) 775-4999

Federation of American
  Health Systems
1111 19th Street, N.W., Suite 402
Washington, DC 20036
(202) 833-3090

Fight for Sight
139 East 57th Street, 7th Floor
New York, NY 10022
(212) 751-1118

Forum for Healthcare Planning
1101 Connecticut Avenue, N.W.,
  Suite 700
Washington, DC 20036
(202) 857-1162

The Gerontological Society
  of America
1411 K Street, N.W., Suite 300
Washington, DC 20005
(202) 393-1411

Gray Panthers
National Office
311 S. Juniper Street, Suite 601
Philadelphia, PA 19107
(215) 545-6555

Group Health Association
  of America
1129 20th Street, N.W., Suite 600
Washington, DC 20036
(202) 778-3200

Guide Dog Foundation for the Blind
371 East Jericho Turnpike
Smithtown, NY 11787
(516) 265-2121

Health and Education
  Resources, Inc.
4733 Bethesda Avenue, Suite 735
Bethesda, MD 20814
(301) 656-3178

Healthcare Financial
  Management Association
2 Westbrook Corporate Center
Westchester, IL 60153
(312) 531-9600

The Healthcare Forum
830 Market Street
San Francisco, CA 94102
(415) 421-8810

Health Insurance Association
  of America
1025 Connecticut Avenue, N.W.,
  Suite 1200
Washington, DC 20036
(202) 223-7780

Home Health Line
Port Republic, MD 20678
(301) 586-0100

Hospital Home Health
67 Peachtree Park Drive, N.E.
Atlanta, GA 30309
(404) 351-4523

Hospital Research
  and Educational Trust
840 North Lake Shore Drive
Chicago, IL 60611
(312) 280-6620

Information Center for
  Individuals with Disabilities, Inc.
20 Park Plaza, Suite 330
Boston, MA 02116
(617) 727-5540

Institute of Gerontology
Wayne State University
71C East Ferry Street,
223 Napp Building
Detroit, MI 48202
(313) 577-2297

Institute on Health and Aging
University of California at San
  Francisco
San Francisco, CA 94143
(415) 476-1000

International Center
  for Social Gerontology
1411 K Street, N.W.,
  Suite 300
Washington, DC 20005
(202) 393-1411

International Federation
  on Aging
1909 K Street, N.W.
Washington, DC 20049
(202) 662-4987

Jewish Association for Services
  for the Aged
40 West 68th Street
New York, NY 10023
(212) 724-3200

Joint Commission on Accreditation
  of Hospitals
875 North Michigan Avenue,
  Suite 2000
Chicago, IL 60611
(312) 642-6061

Lutheran Hospital Association of
  America
Headquarters: Lutheran Hospital
501 10th Avenue
Moline, IL 61265
(309) 757-2611

Lutheran Hospitals and
  Homes Society of America
P.O. Box 2087,
1202 Westrac Drive
Fargo, ND 58107
(701) 293-9053

Medication Education
  for Seniors Citizens
1182 Market Street, Room 204
San Francisco, CA 94102
(415) 558-3767

Mid America Congress on Aging
9400 State Avenue, Room 110
Kansas City, KS 66112
(913) 788-9766

Milbank Memorial Fund
1 East 75th Street
New York, NY 10021
(212) 570-4806

Modern Maturity
4201 Long Beach Boulevard
Long Beach, CA 90807
(213) 427-9611

National Action Forum
  for Older Women
University of Maryland
Center on Aging
College Park, MD 20742
(301) 454-3311

National Alliance of Senior Citizens
2525 Wilson Boulevard
Arlington, VA 22201
(703) 528-4380

National Assembly
  of National Voluntary Health
  and Social Welfare Organizations
1319 F Street, N.W., Suite 601
Washington, DC 20004
(202) 347-2080

National Association for Hearing
  and Speech
10801 Rockville Pike
Rockville, MD 20852
(301) 897-8682

National Association for Home Care
519 C Street, N.E.
Stanton Park
Washington, DC 20002
(202) 547-7424

National Association for Human
  Development
1620 Eye Street, N.W.
Washington, DC 20006
(202) 331-1737

National Association
  for Senior Living Industries
125 Cathedral Street
Annapolis, MD 21401
(301) 263-0991

National Association of Area Agencies
  on Aging
600 Maryland Avenue, S.W., West
  Wing 208
Washington, DC 20024
(202) 484-7520

National Association
  of Mature People
1600 Ninth Street, S.W., Second Floor
Sacramento, CA 95814
(916) 323-4856

National Association of Meal
  Programs
Lutheran Service Society
  of Western Pennsylvania
604 West North Avenue
Pittsburgh, PA 15212
(412) 231-1540

National Association of Nutrition
  and Aging Services Programs
c/o Aging Projects, Inc.
Wiley Building, 104 North Main
Hutchinson, KS 67501
(316) 669-8201

National Association of Older
  American Volunteer
  Program Directors
11481 Bingham Terrace
Reston, VA 22091

National Association of
  Rehabilitation Facilities
5530 Wisconsin Avenue, Suite 955
Washington, DC 20015

National Association of RSVP
  Directors, Inc.
3614 Bryant Avenue South
Minneapolis, MN 55409

National Association of State Units
  on Aging
2033 K Street, N.W., Suite 304
Washington, DC 20006
(202) 785-0707

National Association of Senior
  Companion Project Directors
3225 Lyndale Avenue South
Minneapolis, MN 55408
(612) 827-5641

National Association
  of Social Workers
7981 Eastern Avenue
Silver Spring, MD 20910
(301) 565-0333

National Caucus and Center
  on Black Aged, Inc.
1424 K Street, N.W.,
  Suite 500
Washington, DC 20005
(202) 637-8400

National Council for Homemaker-
  Home Health Aide Service, Inc.
235 Park Avenue South
New York, NY 10003

National Council of Senior Citizens
925 15th Street, N.W.
Washington, DC 20005
(202) 347-8800

National Council on the Aging, Inc.
600 Maryland Avenue, S.W.,
   West Wing 100
Washington, DC 20024
(202) 479-1200

National Dental Association
5506 Connecticut Avenue, N.W.,
   Suite 25
Washington, DC 20015
(202) 244-7555

National Federation of the Blind
1800 Johnson Street
Baltimore, MD 21230
(301) 659-9314

National Geriatrics Society
212 West Wisconsin Avenue, 3rd Floor
Milwaukee, WI 53203
(414) 272-4130

National Health Council, Inc.
622 Third Avenue, 34th Floor
New York, NY 10017-6765
(212) 972-2700

National Health Information
   Clearinghouse
P.O. Box 1133
Washington, DC 20013-1133

National Homecasting Council
235 Park Avenue South, 11th Floor
New York, NY 10003

National Hospice Organization
1901 North Ft. Myer Drive, Suite 307
Arlington, VA 22209
(703) 243-5900

National Interfaith Coalition
   on Aging
P.O. Box 1924
Athens, GA 30603
(404) 353-1331

National Institute of Senior Citizens
c/o National Council on Aging
600 Maryland Avenue, S.W.,
   West Wing 100
Washington, DC 20024
(202) 479-1200

National Institute on Adult
   Day Care
600 Maryland Avenue, S.W.,
   West Wing 100
Washington, DC 20024
(202) 479-1200

National Kidney Foundation
2 Park Avenue
New York, NY 10016
(212) 889-2210

National Mental Health
   Association, Inc.
1021 Prince Street
Alexandria, VA 22314-2971
(703) 684-7722

National Nutrition Consortium, Inc.
1304 Connecticut Avenue, N.W.
Washington, DC 20036
(202) 293-7130

National Pacific/Asian Resource
   Center on Aging
1341 G Street, N.W., Suite 311
Washington, DC 20005

National Parkinson Foundation, Inc.
1501 Ninth Avenue, N.W.
Miami, FL 33136
(305) 547-6666

National Pharmaceutical Association
Howard University
P.O. Box 934
Washington, DC 20059
(202) 328-9229

National Rehabilitation Association
633 S. Washington Street
Alexandria, VA 22314-4193
(703) 836-0850

National Rehabilitation Information
Center
8455 Colesville Road,
Suite 935
Silver Spring, MD 20910
(202) 588-9284

National Safety Council
444 North Michigan Avenue
Chicago, IL 60611
(312) 527-4800

National Senior Citizens Law Center
2025 M Street, N.W.,
Suite 400
Washington, DC 20036
(202) 887-5280

National Stroke Association
1420 Ogden Street
Denver, CO 80218
(303) 839-1992

National Support Center for Families
of the Aging
P.O. Box 245
Swarthmore, PA 19081
(215) 544-5933

National Urban League
Advocacy for the Aged Project
500 East 62nd Street
New York, NY 10021
(212) 310-9000

New Choices for the Best Years
(Formerly 50 Plus)
28 West 23rd Street
New York, NY 10010
(202) 633-4600

New England Gerontological
Association
81 Cutts Road
Durham, NH 03824
(617) 374-0707

Older Women's League
730 11th Street, N.W.,
Suite 300
Washington, DC 20001
(202) 783-6686

Robert Wood Johnson
Foundation
P.O. Box 2316
Princeton, NJ 08540
(609) 452-8701

Salvation Army
799 Bloomfield Avenue
Verona, NJ 07044
(201) 239-0606

Social Security Department/AFL-CIO
815 16th Street, N.W.
Washington, DC 20006
(202) 637-5000

Society for Hospital Planning and
Marketing (AHA)
840 North Lake Shore Drive
Chicago, IL 60611
(312) 280-6086

United Auto Workers
Retired Members Department
8731 East Jefferson
Detroit, MI 48214
(313) 926-5231

United Cancer Council
4010 West 86th Street
Indianapolis, IN 46268
(317) 879-9900

United Hospital Association
2049 Century Park, East, 32nd Floor
Los Angeles, CA 90067
(213) 277-7123

United Parkinson Foundation
360 West Superior Street
Chicago, IL 60610
(312) 664-2344

United Seniors Health Cooperative
1334 G Street, N.W., Suite 500
Washington, DC 20005

United Way of America
701 North Fairfax Street
Alexandria, VA 22314
(703) 836-7100

The Villers Foundation
1334 G Street, N.W.
Washington, DC 20005
(202) 628-3030

Volunteer, The National Center
  Information Service
1111 North 19th Street, Suite 500
Arlington, VA 22209
(703) 276-0542

U.S. Government Agencies

Administration on Aging
Office of Human Development
330 Independence Avenue, S.W.
Washington, DC 20201
(202) 245-0556

Federal Council on Aging
330 Independence Avenue, S.W.
North Building, Room 4620
Washington, DC 20201

National Association of Area Agencies
  on Aging
600 Maryland Avenue, S.W.,
  West Wing 208
Washington, DC 20024
(202) 484-7520

National Association of State Units
  on Aging
2033 K Street, N.W., Suite 304
Washington, DC 20006
(202) 785-0707

National Clearinghouse on Aging
Administration on Aging
330 Independence Avenue, S.W.
DHEW Building, Room 4146
Washington, DC 20201
(202) 245-0995

National Institute on Aging
9000 Rockville Pike
Building 31C, Room 2C02
Bethesda, MD 20892
(301) 496-1752

Office of Human Development
  Services
200 Independence Avenue, S.W.
Washington, DC 20201
(202) 472-7257

Department of Health and Human Services

Disease Prevention and Health
Promotion
Assistant Secretary
(202) 243-7611

Human Development Services
Assistant Secretary
(202) 245-7246

Legislation
Acting Assistant Secretary
(202) 245-7627

Management and Budget
Assistant Secretary
(202) 245-6396

Planning and Evaluation
Assistant Secretary
(202) 245-1858

Public Affairs
Assistant Secretary
(202) 245-1850

Public Health Service
Surgeon General
(202) 245-6467

    Alcohol, Drug Abuse, and Mental
      Health Administration
    Deputy Administrator
    (301) 443-4797

    Centers for Disease Control
    Deputy Director
    (404) 639-3291

    Food and Drug Administration
    Commissioner
    (301) 443-2410

Health Care Financing
Administration
Acting Administrator
(202) 245-6726

Health Resources and Services
Administration
Acting Administrator
(301) 443-2216

National Institute of Health
Director
(301) 496-2433

Social Security Administration
Commissioner
(301) 965-3120

Social Security Administration
Regional Commissioners

    Atlanta: (404) 331-2475

    Boston: (617) 565-1500

    Chicago: (312) 353-5160

    Dallas: (214) 767-3301

    Denver: (303) 844-2388

    Kansas City: (816) 426-2258

    New York: (212) 264-4600

    Philadelphia: (215) 596-6941

    San Francisco: (415) 556-4910

    Seattle: (206) 442-4256

State Units on Aging

ALABAMA

Commission on Aging
State Capitol
Montgomery, AL 36130
(205) 261-5743

ALASKA

Older Alaskans Commission
Department of Administration
P.O. Box C
Juneau, AK 99811-0209
(907) 465-3250

ARIZONA

Aging and Adult Administration
Department of Economic Security
1400 West Washington Street
Phoenix, AZ 85007
(602) 255-4446

ARKANSAS

Office of Aging and Adult Services
Department of Social and
  Rehabilitative Services
Donaghey Building, Suite 1428
7th and Main Streets
Little Rock, AK
(501) 682-2441

CALIFORNIA

Department of Aging
1600 K Street
Sacramento, CA 5814
(916) 322-5290

COLORADO

Aging and Adult Services Division
Department of Social Services
1575 Sherman Street, 10th Floor
Denver, CO 80203-1714
(303) 866-5905

CONNECTICUT

Department on Aging
175 Main Street
Hartford, CT 06106
(203) 566-3238

DELAWARE

Division on Aging
Department of Health and Human
  Services
1901 North Dupont Highway
New Castle, DE 19720
(302) 421-6791

DISTRICT OF COLUMBIA

Office on Aging
1424 K Street, N.W., 2nd Floor
Washington, DC 20005
(202) 724-5626

FLORIDA

Program Office of Aging Services
Department of Health and
  Rehabilitation Services
1317 Winewood Boulevard
Tallahassee, FL 32301
(904) 488-8922

GEORGIA

Office of Aging
878 Peachtree Street, N.E.,
  Room 632
Atlanta, GA 30309
(404) 894-5333

GUAM

Public Health and
  Social Services
Government of Guam
Agana, Guam 96910

HAWAII

Executive Office
  of Aging
Office of the Governor
335 Merchant Street,
  Room 241
Honolulu, HI 96813
(808) 548-2593

IDAHO

Office on Aging
Statehouse,
  Room 108
Boise, ID 83720
(208) 334-3833

ILLINOIS

Department of Aging
421 East Capitol Avenue
Springfield, IL 62701
(217) 785-2870

INDIANA

Department of Aging and Community
  Services
251 North Illinois Street, Box 7083
Indianapolis, IN 46207
(317) 232-7006

IOWA

Commission on Aging
914 Grand Avenue
Jewett Building, Suite 236
Des Moines, IA 50319
(515) 281-5187

KANSAS

Department on Aging
122 South Docking State Office Bldg.
915 Southwest Harrison
Topeka, KS 66612
(913) 296-4986

KENTUCKY

Division for Aging Services
Department of Resources
CHR Building, 6th Floor
275 East Main Street
Frankfort, KY 40621
(502) 564-6930

LOUISIANA

Office of Elderly Affairs
P.O. Box 80374
Baton Rouge, LA 70898
(504) 925-1700

MAINE

Bureau of Maine's Elderly
Department of Human
  Services
Statehouse, Station 11
Augusta, ME 04333
(207) 289-2561

MARYLAND

Office on Aging
State Office Building
301 West Preston Street,
  Room 1004
Baltimore, MD 21201
(301) 225-1100

MASSACHUSETTS

Department of Elder Affairs
38 Chauncy Street
Boston, MA 02111
(617) 727-7750

MICHIGAN

Office of Services to the Aging
P.O. Box 30026
Lansing, MI 48909
(517) 373-8230

MINNESOTA

Board on Aging
Human Services Building,
  4th Floor
444 Layayett Road
St. Paul, MN 55155-3843
(612) 296-2544

MISSISSIPPI

Council on Aging
301 West Pearl Street
Jackson, MS 39203-3092
(601) 949-2070

MISSOURI

Division on Aging
Department of Social Services
P.O. Box 1337
2701 West Main
Jefferson City, MO 65102
(314) 751-3082

MONTANA

Community Service Division
P.O. Box 8005
Helena, MT 59604
(406) 444-3865

NEBRASKA

Department on Aging
P.O. Box 95044
301 Centennial Mall South
Lincoln, NB 68509
(402) 471-2306

NEVADA

Division on Aging
Department of Human Resources
505 East King Street
Kinkead Building,
  Room 101
Carson City, NV 89710
(702) 885-4210

PENNSYLVANIA

Department of Aging
231 State Street
Harrisburg, PA 17101-1195
(717) 783-1550

PUERTO RICO

Gericulture Commission
Department of Social Services
P.O. Box 11398
Santurce, PR 00910
(809) 721-3141 or 722-0225

RHODE ISLAND

Department of Elderly Affairs
79 Washington Street
Providence, RI 02903
(401) 277-2858

AMERICAN SAMOA

Territorial Administration on Aging
Office of the Governor
Pago Pago, Samoa 96799
011 (684) 633-1252

SOUTH CAROLINA

Commission on Aging
400 Arbor Lake Drive, Suite B-500
Columbia, SC 29223
(803) 735-0210

SOUTH DAKOTA

Office of Adult Services and Aging
700 Governor's Drive, Kneip Bldg.
Pierre, SD 57501
(605) 773-3656

TENNESSEE

Commission on Aging
706 Church Street,
  Suite 201
535 Church Street
Nashville, TN 37219
(615) 741-2056

TEXAS

Department of Aging
P.O. Box 12786,
  Capitol Station
1949 IH 35, South
Austin, TX 78741-3702
(512) 444-2727

TRUST TERRITORY OF THE
PACIFIC

Office of Elderly Programs
Community Development
  Division
Government of TTPI
Saipan, Mariana Islands 96950
9335 or 9336

UTAH

Division of Aging
  and Adult Services
Department of Social Services
120 North 200 West
Salt Lake City, UT 84103
(801) 538-3910

VERMONT

Office on Aging
103 South Main Street
Waterbury, VT 05676
(802) 241-2400

NEW HAMPSHIRE

Division of Elderly and
  Adult Services
6 Hazen Drive
Concord, NH 03301
(603) 271-4394

NEW JERSEY

Division on Aging
Department of Community Affairs
CN-807
Trenton, NJ 08625
(609) 292-4833

NEW MEXICO

State Agency on Aging
224 East Palace Avenue,
  4th Floor
La Villa Rivera Building
Santa Fe, NM 87501
(505) 827-7640

NEW YORK

Office for the Aging
New York State Plaza
Agency Building 2
Albany, NY 12223
(518) 474-4425

NORTH CAROLINA

Division on Aging
1985 Umpstead Drive
Kirby Building
Raleigh, NC 27603
(919) 733-3983

NORTH DAKOTA

Aging Services
Department of Human Service
State Capitol Building
Bismark, ND 58505
(701) 224-2577

NORTHERN MARIANA
ISLANDS

Office on Aging
Department of Community and
  Cultural Affairs
Civic Center, Susupe
Saipan, Northern Mariana Islands
  96950
9411 or 9732

OHIO

Department on Aging
50 West Broad Street, 9th Floor
Columbus, OH 43266-0501
(614) 466-5500

OKLAHOMA

Special Unit on Aging
Department of Human Services
P.O. Box 25352
Oklahoma City, OK 73125
(405) 521-2281

OREGON

Senior Services Division
313 Public Service Building
Salem, OR 97310
(503) 378-4728

VIRGINIA

Department on Aging
700 East Franklin Street, 10th Floor
Richmond, VA 23219-2327
(804) 225-2271

VIRGIN ISLANDS

Commission on Aging
6F Havensight Mall-Charlotte Amalie
St. Thomas, VI 00801
(809) 774-5884

WASHINGTON

Bureau of Aging and Adult Services
Department of Social and Health
  Services
OB-44A
Olympia, WA 98504
(206) 753-2502

WEST VIRGINIA

Commission on Aging
Holly Grove, State Capitol
Charleston, WV 25305
(304) 348-3317

WISCONSIN

Bureau of Aging
Division of Community Services
217 S. Hamilton Street, Suite 300
Madison, WI 53703
(608) 266-2536

WYOMING

Commission on Aging
Hathaway Building, Room 139
Cheyenne, WY 82002-0710
(307) 777-7986

List of
Recommended Readings

Allen, John B. "Housing for the Elderly." *Investor Outlook*, Second Quarter, 1986.

American Association of Retired Persons. *A Profile of Older Americans*. Washington, D.C.: AARP, 1985.

American Association of Retired Persons. *Your Home, Your Choice: A Workbook for Older People and Their Families*. Washington, D.C.: AARP, 1984.

American Hospital Association. *AHA Guide to the Health Care Field*. Chicago: AHA, 1986.

American Hospital Association. *Health Promotion for Older Adults II: Effective Ideas for $5000*. Teleconference held May 29, 1986. Chicago: AHA, 1986.

American Hospital Association. Hospital Research and Educational Trust. "1985 Hospital Costs and Utilization." *Economic Trends*, Spring 1986.

American Hospital Association. Hospital Research and Educational Trust. *Emerging Trends in Aging and Long-Term Care Services*. Chicago: HRET, 1986.

American Hospital Association. *Hospital Strategies and Resources for Communicating with Seniors*. Chicago: AHA, 1985.

American Hospital Association. Hospital Research and Educational Trust. *The Hospitals Role in Caring for the Elderly: Leadership Issues*. Chicago: HRET, 1982.

Andersen, Arthur, & Co. *Health Care in the 1990s: Trends and Strategies 1984*. New York: Arthur Andersen, 1984.

Andersen, Ronald, LuAnn Aday, and Meei-shia Chen. "Health Status and Medical Care Utilization." *Health Affairs*, Spring 1986.

Anderson, Gerald F. "Data Watch." *Health Affairs*, Fall 1985.

Anderson, Howard J. "Home Care Providers' Business Expanded Rapidly During 1985." *Modern Healthcare*, June 6, 1986.

265

Anderson, Howard J., and Mark F. Baldwin. "U.S. Healthcare Spending Undergoes Smallest 1-Year Increase in 20 Years." *Modern Healthcare*, August 15, 1986.

Arnett, Ross H., et al. "Projections of Health Care Spending to 1990." *Healthcare Financing Review*, Spring 1986.

Atkins, Lawrence G. "The Economic Status of the Oldest Old." *Milbank Memorial Fund Quarterly*, Spring 1985.

Avorn, Jerome L. "Medicine, Health, and the Geriatric Transformation." *Daedalus*, Winter 1986.

Baginsk, Yvonne. "Marketing Home Care to the Doctors." *Caring*, September 1985.

Baldwin, Mark F. "GAO Study Recommends Reduced Medicare Payments to Prepaid Plans." *Modern Healthcare*, August 1, 1986.

Baldwin, Mark F. "Hospital Leaders Fear First-Year Profits Will Trigger Medicare Payment Freeze." *Modern Healthcare*, March 14, 1986.

Baldwin, Mark F. "Medicare Payments Increased 0.5 Percent." *Modern Healthcare*, September 12, 1986.

Baldwin, Mark F. "Prospective Pricing May Survive Extensive Reform of Medicare." *Modern Healthcare*, August 15, 1986.

Bentkover, Judith, et al. "The Future of Medicare." *New England Journal of Medicine*, March 13, 1986.

Berk, S.E. "Commentary: DRGs, Incentives, Hospitals, and Physicians." *Health Affairs*, Winter 1985.

Bernstein, Roger M., and Margrit Stolz Bernstein. "Medicare Bill Jeopardizes Middle-class Assets." *Miami Herald*, June 26, 1988.

Bernstein Research. *The Future of Health Care Delivery in America*. New York: Sanford Bernstein & Co., 1988.

Birren, James E., and K. Warner Schaie. *Handbook of the Psychology of Aging*. New York: Van Nostrand Reinhold, 1977.

Bisbee, Gerald E., and Mark J. Simon. *Long-Term Care Industry*. New York: Kidder Peabody Co., October 1985.

Bishop, Christine E. "Living Arrangement Choices of Elderly Singles: Effect of Income and Disability." *Health Care Financing Review*, Spring 1986.

"Blues Plans Cover Home Care as Economy Measure." *Modern Healthcare*, August 16, 1986.

Brody, Elaine M. "Parent Care as a Normative Family Stress." *The Gerontologist*, February 1985.

Brody, Stanley J., and Nancy A. Persily. *Hospitals and the Aged: The New Old Market*. Rockville, Maryland: Aspen Systems Corporation, 1984.

California Health Facilities Commission. *Guide to California Health Care Costs*. Sacramento: State of California, December 1985.

Callahan, Daniel. "Adequate Health Care and an Aging Society: Are They Morally Compatible?" *Daedalus*, Winter 1986.

Carlson, Elliot. "Is Our Care System Killing Us?" *Modern Maturity*, April/May 1984.

Carlson, Eugene. "New Study Looks at the State of Nation's 'Old-Old' Citizens." *Wall Street Journal*, August 5, 1986.

Caserta, Michael S., et al. "Caregivers to Dementia Patients: The Utilization of Community Services." Unpublished paper.

"Catastrophic Illness Options Considered." *Modern Healthcare*, September 12, 1986.

Center for Health Studies. *The Aging Population: Implications for Hospitals*. Nashville: Center for Health Studies, May 1982.

Coile, Russell C. "Healthcare Industry Outlook: Macrotrends for 1990." Unpublished paper, 1986.

Collins, Glenn. "More Women Work Longer." *New York Times*, April 3, 1986.

"Commercial Insurers Will Win—Goldsmith." *Modern Healthcare*, April 25, 1986.

"CON Laws Cause Higher Home Care Costs—FTC." *Modern Healthcare*, April 11, 1986.

Conference Board. Consumer Research Center. *Midlife and Beyond: The $800 Billion Over-Fifty Market*. New York: Conference Board, 1985.

Coombs Ficke, Susan. *An Orientation to the Older Americans Act*. Washington, D.C.: National Association of State Units on Aging, July 1985.

Corey, E. Raymond. "Marketing Strategy—An Overview." Boston: Harvard Business School, 1978.

CRLA Foundation. "IHSS Vital to Long-Term Care." *Long-Term Care Reporter*, November/December 1985.

Cromwell, Jerry, and Philip Burstein. "Physician Losses from Medicare and Medicaid Discounts: How Real Are They?" *Health Care Financing Review*, Summer 1985.

Davidson, Joe. "Reagan's Efforts to Ease Financial Burdens of Catastrophic Illness to Focus on Elderly." *Wall Street Journal*, February 6, 1986.

Davis, Karen. "Aging and the Health Care System: Economic and Structural Issues." *Daedalus*, Winter 1986.

Davis, Karen. *Health Implications of Aging in America*. Baltimore, Maryland: Johns Hopkins University, 1983.

"Dispelling The Myths." *National Association for Senior Living Industries News*, May/June 1986.

"Drug Makers See Opportunity in Rise of Psychogeriatrics as Baby Boom Generation Ages." *Chemical Marketing News*, June 4, 1986.

"Durenberger Proposes Partial Payment for New Treatment." *Modern Healthcare*, June 6, 1986.

Dychtwald, Ken. *Wellness and Health Promotion for the Elderly*. Rockville, Maryland: Aspen Systems Corporation, 1986.

Ellwood, Deborah A. "Medicare Risk Contracting." *Health Affairs*, Spring 1986.

Ellwood, Paul M., and Barbara A. Paul. *Here Come the Supermeds*. Excelsior, Minnesota: InterStudy, n.d.

Ellwood, Paul M., and Linda Krane Ellwein. "Physician Glut Will Force Hospitals to Look Outward." *Hospitals*, January 16, 1981.

Elwell, Frank. "The Effects of Ownership on Institution Services." *The Gerontologist*, February 1984.

Enthoven, Alain. "Health Tax Policy Mismatch." *Health Affairs*, Winter 1985.

Evashwick, Connie J., Janice Neg, and James Siemon. "*Case Management: Issues for Hospitals*." Chicago: The Hospital Research and Educational Trust, 1985.

Evashwick, Connie J., and William Read. "Hospitals and LTC: Options, Alternatives, Implications." *Healthcare Financial Management*, June 1984.

Eversen, Laura H., and Cynthia L. Polich. *The Future of Medicare and HMOs*. Excelsior, Minnesota: InterStudy, 1985.

Eversen, Laura H., et al. *The 1985 Medicare and HMOs Data Book*. Excelsior, Minnesota: InterStudy, 1985.

"Farsighted Developers Build for the Elderly." *San Francisco Chronicle*, May 27, 1986.

Ferrara, Peter J. *Averting the Medicare Crisis: Health IRAs*. Washington, D.C.: Cato Institute, October 31, 1985.

Ferrara, Peter J. "Don't Entrust Catastrophic Coverage to Medicare." *Wall Street Journal*, March 12, 1986.

Firman, James P. "Health Care Cooperatives: Innovations for Older People." *Health Affairs*, Winter 1985.

Fishman, Linda. "Home Health Under Medicare." *Long-Term Care Reporter*, November/December 1985.

Florida Power and Light Company. *Impact for the 1980s*. Miami: FPL, 1986.

Flower, Joe. "Coming of Age." *Healthcare Forum*, November/December 1985.

Flynn, Cynthia B., et al. "The Redistribution of America's Older Population: Major National Migration Patterns for Three Census Decades, 1960–1980." *The Gerontologist*, June 1985.

Francese, Peter K. "Women as Healthcare Consumers." *Healthcare Forum*, January/February 1986.

Freedman, Alix M. "Nursing Homes Try New Approach in Caring for Alzheimer's Victims." *Wall Street Journal*, September 26, 1986.

Freudenheim, Milt. "Help in Caring for the Elderly." *New York Times*, July 1, 1986.

Freudenheim, Milt. "Hospice Care As an Option." *New York Times*, February 4, 1986.

Freudenheim, Milt. "Medical Costs Continue to Surge; Evasion of Controls Held as Cause." *New York Times*, July 26, 1986.

Fritschner, Sarah. "The Ageless Problems of Nutrition." *Washington Post*, December 3, 1981.

Fuchs, Victor. *How We Live*. Cambridge: Harvard University Press, 1983.

Fuerbringer, Jonathan. "Senate Panel Votes $3 Billion Savings in Medicare." *New York Times*, July 23, 1986.

Ginsburg, Paul B., and Marilyn Moon. "An Introduction to the Medicare Financing Problem." *Milbank Memorial Fund Quarterly*, Spring, 1984.

Golden, Patrica M. *Charting the Nation's Health*. Washington, D.C.: Government Printing Office, August 1985.

Goldsmith, Jeff. "2036: A Health Care Odyssey." *Hospitals*, May 5, 1986.

Gordon, William. "Graying of Jersey Spurs Innovation in Housing Options." Newark, New Jersey, *Star-Ledger*, April 27, 1986.

Graham, Judith. "New York Shows Hospital Preferences." *Modern Healthcare*, July 4, 1986.

Grana, John M., and David B. McCallum, eds. *The Impact of Technology on Long-Term Health Care*. Millwood, Virginia: Center for Health Affairs, Project HOPE, 1986.

Grant, William D., and Marcia R. Smith. "Discharge Planning and Discharge Criteria in Adult Day Care Programs: A National Survey." Oklahoma City: Oklahoma University Health Sciences Center, 1986.

Greenhouse, Steven. "Health Plans Are Feeling a Little Peaked." *New York Times*, August 24, 1986.

Greer, David S., and Vincent Mor. "How Medicare Is Altering the Hospice Movement." *Hastings Center Report*, October 1985.

Grimaldi, Paul L. "How Major Regulations Strive to Ensure Quality Care in Nursing." *Healthcare Financial Management*, September 1984.

Guterman, Stuart, and Allen Dobson. "Impact of the Medicare Prospective Payment System for Hospitals." *Health Care Financing Review*, Spring 1986.

Hagestad, Gunhild O. "The Aging Society as a Context for Family Life." *Daedalus*, Winter 1986.

Haglund, Claudia L., et al. "Out-of-Plan Use by Medicare Enrollees in a Risk-Sharing Health Maintenance Organization." *Health Care Financing Review*, Winter 1985.

Harrington, Charlene, et al. *Long Term Care of the Elderly*. Beverly Hills, SAGE Publications, 1985.

Harrington, Charlene, and James H. Swan. "Medicaid Nursing Home Reimbursement Policies, Rates, and Expenditures." *Health Care Financing Review*, Fall 1984.

Harvard University. Division of Health Policy Research and Education. *Medicare: Coming of Age—A Proposal Reform*. Boston: Harvard Business School, 1986.

"Healthcare Analysts See Slower Growth for Beverly." *Modern Healthcare*, April 11, 1986.

"Health-Care Financing Info." *Nursing Homes*, March/April 1985.

Health Insurance Association of America. *Long-Term Care: The Challenge to Society.* Washington, D.C.: HIAA, 1984.

"Help for Women Old and Young." *New York Times,* May 29, 1986.

Hiatt, Lorraine G., "Architecture for the Aged: Design for Living." *Inland Architect,* November/December 1977.

Hiatt, Lorraine G., "Disorientation Is More Than a State of Mind." *Nursing Homes,* July/August 1980.

Hoffer, William. "Making Social Security Private." *Nation's Business,* July 1986.

Hollie, Pamela G. "Corporate Elder Care." *New York Times,* June 22, 1986.

"Hospital Occupancy Rate Hits a Record Low at 63.6 Percent." *Modern Healthcare,* April 25, 1986.

"IG Recommends Indirect Payments Be Reconsidered." *Modern Healthcare,* June 6, 1986.

Iglehart, John K. "Congress, Public Policy, and the Future: A Conversation with Bill Aradison." *Health Affairs,* Winter 1985.

Inguanzo, Joe M., and Mark Harju. "How Do Consumers Receive Local Health Care Information?" *Hospitals,* April 1, 1985.

Jazwiecki, Tom. "How States Pay for Long-Term Care Facility Services." *Healthcare Financial Management,* April 1984.

Jensen, Joyce. "Consumers Who Notice Ads Recall Messages." *Modern Healthcare,* April 11, 1986.

Jensen, Joyce. "More Consumers Are Willing to Pay a Higher Price for Quality Healthcare." *Modern Healthcare,* August 15, 1986.

Jensen, Joyce. "Trust in Doctor Deters Elderly from Seeing Other Providers." *Modern Healthcare,* April 25, 1986.

Jensen, Joyce, and Ned Miklovic. "Consumers Turn to Yellow Pages When Making Healthcare Choices." *Modern Healthcare,* June 20, 1986.

Jernigan, James A. "Update on Drugs and the Elderly." *American Family Physician,* April 1984.

Johnson, Donald E.L. "Hospitals Expected to Acquire Larger Share of Long-Term Care." *Modern Healthcare,* August 15, 1986.

Johnson, Donald E.L. "Patient's Healthcare Needs Dictate Who Influences Choice of Providers." *Modern Healthcare,* May 9, 1986.

Keeler, Emmett B., Robert Kane, and David Solomon. "Short- and Long-Term Residents of Nursing Homes." *Medical Care,* March 1981.

Kethley, Alice J., and Martha K. Parker. *A National Inventory of Services to Help Families Care for Older Family Members.* Excelsior, Minnesota: InterStudy, 1984.

Keyfitz, Nathan. "Population Appearances and Demographic Reality." *Population and Development Review,* March 1980.

Kiester, Edward Jr. "Young vs. Old—The War We Must Never Allow to Happen." *50 Plus*, August 1986.

Knickman, James R., and Nelda McCall. "A Prepaid Managed Approach to Long-Term Care." *Health Affairs*, Spring 1986.

Koren, Mary Jane. "Home Care—Who Cares?" *New England Journal of Medicine*, April 3, 1986.

Kotler, Philip. *Marketing Management: Analysis, Planning, and Control.* Englewood Cliffs, New Jersey: Prentice-Hall, 1984.

Langer, Judith. *Consumers in Transition: In-Depth Investigations of Changing Lifestyles.* New York: American Management Associations, 1982.

LeRoy, Lauren, John K. Iglehart, and Deborah A. Ellwood. "Trends in Health Manpower." *Health Affairs*, Winter 1985.

Lessman, Karen S. "Addressing the Needs of the Frail Elderly." *Hospital Forum*, July/August 1980.

Leutz, W.N., Jay N. Greenberg, Ruby Abrahams, Jeffrey Prottus, Larry M. Diamond, and Leonard Gruenberg. *Changing Health Care for an Aging Society.* Lexington, Massachusetts: D.C. Heath & Company, 1985.

Levit, Katharine R., et al. "National Health Expenditures, 1984." *Health Care Financing Review*, Fall 1985.

Levit, Katharine R. "Personal Health Care Expenditures by State: 1966-82." *Health Care Financing Review*, Summer 1985.

Laventhol & Horwath. *Lifecare Retirement Center Industry 1985.* Philadelphia: Laventhol & Horwath, 1985.

Liu, Korbin, and Kenneth G. Manton. "The Characteristics and Utilization Pattern of an Admission Cohort of Nursing Home Patients." *The Gerontologist*, February 1983.

Liu, Korbin, Kenneth G. Manton, and Barbara Marzetta Liu. "Home Care Expenses for the Disabled Elderly." *Health Care Financing Review*, Winter 1985.

Liu, Korbin, and Yuko Palesch. "The Nursing Home Population: Different Perspectives and Implications for Policy." *Health Care Financing Review*, December 1981.

Logan, John R. "The Graying of the Suburbs." *Aging*, June/July 1984.

Longman, Phillip. "Justice Between Generations." *Atlantic Monthly*, June 1985.

Louis Harris and Associates. *"Aging in the Eighties: America in Transition.* Washington, D.C.: National Council on the Aging, 1981.

Lubitz, James, Gerald Reily, and Marilyn Newton. "Outcomes of Surgery in the Medicare Aged Population: Mortality After Surgery." *Health Care Financing Review*, Summer 1985.

Lubitz, James, and Ronald Prihoda. "The Use and Costs of Medicare Services in the Last 2 Years." *Health Care Financing Review*, Spring 1984.

Mallory, James M., and David B. Skinner. "Medicare on the Critical List." *Harvard Business Review*, November/December 1984.

Maloney, Susan K., Barbara Fallon, and Clarissa K. Wittenberg. *Aging and Health Promotion: Market Research for Public Education—Executive Summary.* Washington, D.C.: ODPHP, May 1984.

Manton, Kenneth G., and Korbin Liu. *The Future Growth of the Long-Term Care Population:* Washington, D.C.: NCHS, March 1984.

Marriott Corporation. *The Art of Lifecare.* Bethesda, Maryland: Marriott, 1985.

Mastalish, Raymond C. "Reaching The Nation's Elderly Through the Network of Aging." *National Association for Senior Living Industries News,* May/June 1986.

McCulloch, Catherine A. "A Hospital Planning Response to the Geriatric Imperative." *Health Care Strategic Management,* November 1983.

McIntosh, Alison C. "Low Fertility and Liberal Democracy in Western Europe." *Population and Development Review,* June 1981.

McMillan, Alma, James Lubitz, and Marilyn Newton. "Trends in Physician Assignment Rates for Medicare Services, 1968–84." *Health Care Financing Review,* Winter 1985.

"Medicare Could Go Broke in 1990s." *San Francisco Chronicle,* April 1, 1986.

Menken, Jane. "Age Fertility: How Late Can You Wait?" *Demography,* November 1985.

Merrill, Jefferey C., and Richard J. Wassermann. "Growth in National Expenditures: Additional Analyses." *Health Affairs,* Winter 1985.

"Miami's Elderly: The Future of Health Care?" *Hospitals,* March 20, 1986.

Miner, Steven. "Outpatient Services for the Disabled." *Aging,* 1985.

Moody, Harry R. "Education in an Aging Society." *Daedalus,* Winter 1986.

"National Medical Care Spending." *Health Affairs,* Fall 1985.

"A New Alternative in North Beach for Frail Elderly." *San Francisco Examiner,* May 12, 1986.

Newcomer, Robert, and Robyn Stone. "Board and Care Housing: Expansion and Improvement Needed." *Generations,* Summer 1985.

Nimer, Daniel A. "Meet the Competition? Why Should I?" *Healthcare Forum,* July/August 1986.

Nimer, Daniel A. "On the Pricing of Joy Perfume, Mercedes, Hospital Services, Etc...." *Health Care Forum,* May/June 1986.

Oji-McNair, Kathleen. "A Cost Analysis of Hospice versus Non-Hospice Care: Positioning Characteristics for Marketing a Hospice." *Health Marketing Quarterly,* Summer 1985.

Oram, Donna M. "The Challenge of Marketing Professional Services." *Caring,* September 1985.

Ostroff, Jeffery M. *Accessing Mature (Age 55 +) Health Care Consumers Through Caregivers and Corporations.* Proceedings of the Academy for Health Services Marketing, 1986.

Otten, Alan L. "Decision Makers Often Fail to Spot Key Changes Behind the Statistics." *Wall Street Journal*, December 6, 1985.

Ouslander, Joseph G. "Drug Therapy in the Elderly." *Annals of Internal Medicine*, December 1981.

Palmer, John L., and Stephanie G. Gould. "The Economic Consequences of an Aging Society." *Daedalus*, Winter 1986.

Pear, Robert. "A Slight Rise Seen in Medicare Rate Paid to Hospitals." *New York Times*, May 29, 1986.

Pear, Robert. "Curbs on Medicaid Being Considered." *New York Times*, July 13, 1986.

Pear, Robert. "Reagan Seeking Fixed Medicare Fees for Doctors." *New York Times*, December 7, 1985.

Pear, Robert. "President to Seek Medicare Changes." *New York Times*, November 24, 1984.

Pegels, C.C. *Health Care and the Elderly*. Rockville, Maryland: Aspen Systems Corporation, 1981.

"Pepper's Bill Would Create Part C Medicare Coverage." *Modern Healthcare*, April 11, 1986.

Peters, Joseph P. *A Strategic Planning Process for Hospitals* Chicago: American Hospital Publishing, 1985.

Pifer, Alan, and D. Lydia Bronte. "Introduction: Squaring the Pyramid." *Daedalus*, Winter 1986.

"Pill Colors Confuse Elderly." *New England Journal of Medicine*, January 19, 1984.

Pomeranz, William, and Steven Rosenberg. "Developing an Adult Day-Care Center." *Journal of Long-Term Care Administration*, Spring 1985.

Porter, Michael E. "Note on the Structural Analysis of Industries." Boston: Harvard Business School, 1975.

Potetz, Lisa, and Thomas Buchbeger. "Medicare's Transition to National Payment Rates: Effects on Hospitals." *Health Affairs*, Winter 1985.

"Pre-Screening." *Long-Term Care Reporter*, November/December 1985.

Prisuta, Robert H. "Age As a Predictor of Demographic Status, Attitudes and Behavior Among Older Persons." Unpublished paper.

"Private Catastrophic Plans Pushed by Conservatives." *Modern Healthcare*, July 4, 1986.

Project HOPE. *Health Prospects: 1983–2003*. Millwood, Virginia: Project HOPE, 1985.

Project SHARE. *How-to Manual on Providing Respite Care for Family Caregivers*. Rockville, Maryland: Project SHARE, May 1985.

Promoting Health/Preventing Disease: Public Health Service Implementation Plans for Attaining the Objectives for the Nation. Washington, D.C.: Government Printing Office, October 1983.

"Proposals Regulating Nursing Home Care May Follow Report." *Modern Healthcare*, June 6, 1986.

Relman, Arnold S., and Uwe E. Reinhardt. "Debating For-Profit Health Care." *Health Affairs*, Summer 1986.

Riche, Martha Farnsworth. "The Nursing Home Dilemma." *American Demographics*, October 1985.

Richman, Dan, and Mark F. Baldwin. "Government Spending Cuts Force HMOs to Walk Payment Tightrope." *Modern Healthcare*, September 12, 1986.

Richter, Todd B. *Gone with the Wind.* New York: Morgan Stanley, January 31, 1986.

Riles, Gerald, et al. "Changes in Distribution of Medicare Expenditures Among Aged Enrollees, 1962–82." *Healthcare Financing Review*, Spring 1986.

Roessing, Walter. "Aging Well." *Sky Magazine*, March 1986.

Rogers, David, "Budget Measure to Affect Costs for Employers." *Wall Street Journal*, March 23, 1986.

Rohrer, Robert L., and Robert Bibb. *Product Segmentation and Marketing Challenges in the Senior Housing Industry.* Annapolis, Maryland: National Association for Senior Living Industries, 1986.

Rudensky, Maria. "Case Managers May Boost Admissions." *Modern Healthcare*, August 1986.

Sabin, Sandy. "Rehab Program's Marketing Plan Was Tailored to Fit." *Nursing & Health Care*, May 1985.

"Sasser Bill Would Expand Coverage Under Medicare." *Modern Healthcare*, July 18, 1986.

Scanlon, William J., and Judith Feder. "The Long-Term Care Marketplace: An Overview." *Healthcare Financial Management*, January 1984.

Schoen, Robert, et al. "Marriage and Divorce in Twentieth Century American Cohorts." *Demography*, February 1985.

Segal, Wayne M. "A Hospital Rehabilitation Center: Preparation for Going Home." *Aging*, 1985.

Shahoda, Teri. "Demand for Certain Rehab Services Is on the Upswing." *Hospitals*, June 1, 1985.

Shepherd, Paul, and G. Richard Ambrosius. *Aging Is....Just a Series of Beginnings.* Sioux Falls, South Dakota: Phoenix Systems, 1985.

Sherwood, Sylvia, John N. Morris, and Hirsch S. Ruchlin. "Alternative Paths to Long-Term Care: Nursing Home Geriatric Day Hospital, Senior Center, and Domiciliary Care Options." *American Journal of Public Health*, January 1986.

Siegel, Jacob S., and Cynthia M. Taeuber. "Demographic Perspectives on the Long-Lived Society." *Daedalus*, Winter 1986.

Sims, William B. "Financing Strategies for Long-Term Care Facilities." *Healthcare Financial Management*, March 1984.

Sloane, Leonard. "Lifetime Care in Retirement." *New York Times*, June 14, 1986.

Snyder, Lorraine Hiatt. "Environmental Changes for Socialization." *Journal of Nursing Administration*, January 1978.

"A Special News Report on People and Their Jobs in Offices, Fields, and Factories." *Wall Street Journal*, August 12, 1986.

Steinberg, R.M., and G.W. Carter. *Case Management and the Elderly*. Lexington, Massachusetts: Lexington Books, 1983.

Stewart, Natalie. "Marketing Tools and Methods for Small Home Health Agencies." *Caring*, September 1985.

Stone, Robyn, Gail Lee Cafferata, and Judith Sangl. *Caregivers of the Frail Elderly: A National Profile*. National Center for Health Services Research and Health Care Technology Assessment, 1986.

Sullivan, Ronald. "At New York Hospitals, Empty Beds." *New York Times*, April 20, 1986.

Sulvetta, Margaret B., and John Holahan. "Cost and Case-Mix Differences Between Hospital-Based and Freestanding Nursing Homes." *Health Care Financing Review*, Spring 1986.

"A Summary of Veterans Administration Benefits." Veterans Administration, 1984.

Super, Kari E. "Hospitals Are Beginning to Focus on Services for Older Patients." *Modern Healthcare*, April 11, 1986.

Super, Kari E. "Two Tennessee Hospitals Joining Consortium That Provides Referral Service to Elderly." *Modern Health Care*, March 28, 1986.

Tedesco, Janet A., and DeWayne L. Oberlander. *Adult Day Care*. Chicago: Hospital Research and Educational Trust, 1983.

Tedesco, Janet A., and Mary E. Longe. *Health Promotion and Wellness*. Chicago: Hospital Research and Educational Trust, 1984.

Tehan, Claire. "Has Success Spoiled Hospice?" *Hastings Center Report*, October 1985.

Ting, Harold M. "New Directions in Nursing Home and Home Healthcare Marketing." *Healthcare Financial Management*, May 1984.

Tydings, Joseph D. "Legislative Report." *National Association for Senior Living Industries News*, May/June 1986.

U.S. Bureau of the Census. *America in Transition: An Aging Society*. Current Population Reports, Series P-23, No. 128. Washington, D.C.: Government Printing Office, 1983.

U.S. Bureau of the Census. *Marital Status and Living Arrangements: March 1984*. Washington, D.C.: Government Printing Office, 1985.

U.S. Congress, Office of Technology Assessment. *Technology and Aging in America*. Washington, D.C.: Government Printing Office, June 1985.

U.S. National Center for Health Statistics. *Charting the Nation's Health: Trends Since 1960*. Washington, D.C.: Government Printing Office, August 1985.

U.S. National Center for Health Statistics. *Current Estimates from the National Health Interview Survey: United States, 1982*. Vital and Health Statistics, Series 10, No. 150. Hyattsville, Maryland: NCHS, September 1985.

U.S. National Center for Health Statistics. *Health Characteristics of Persons with Chronic Activity Limitation: United States, 1979*. Vital and Health Statistics, Series 10, No. 137. Hyattsville, Maryland: NCHS, December 1981.

U.S. National Center for Health Statistics. *Health, United States, 1985*. Washington, D.C.: Government Printing Office, December 1985.

U.S. ODPHP. *Health Promotion and Disease Prevention for Older Americans: Communication Strategy Statement*. Draft, December 5, 1984.

"U.S. Says Hospitals Profit from Medicare." *San Francisco Chronicle*, July 14, 1986.

U.S. Senate Special Committee on Aging. *Aging America/Trends and Projections*. Washington, D.C.: Government Printing Office, 1986.

Urbonya, Tim. "Room for Profits in Senior Housing?" *San Francisco Examiner*, June 8, 1986.

Veterans Administration. *Caring for the Older Veteran*. Washington, D.C.: Government Printing Office, July 1984.

Vladeck, Bruce. "America's Hospitals." *Health Affairs*, Summer 1986.

Vogel, R.J., and H.C. Palmer. *Long-Term Care: Perspectives from Research and Demonstrations*. Rockville, Maryland: Aspen Systems Corporation, 1985.

Waldholz, Michael. "Most Hospitals Quickly Learn to Be Profitable." *Wall Street Journal*, August 28, 1985.

Waldo, Daniel R., and Helen C. Lazenby. "Demographic Characteristics and Health Care Use and Expenditures by the Aged in the United States: 1977–1984. *Health Care Financing Review*, Fall 1984.

Wallace, Cynthia. "HFCA Nominee Advocates Capitation." *Modern Healthcare*, April 25, 1986.

Wallace, Cynthia. "House May Delay Capital Payment Plan." *Modern Healthcare*, April 25, 1986

Weiler, Philip G. "Estimating Need for Adult Day Health Care." *Health Services Quarterly*, Spring 1985.

Weissert, William G. "Estimating the Long-Term Care Population: Prevalence Rates and Selected Characteristics." *Health Care Financing Review*, Summer 1985.

"What Do Patients Really Want?" *Healthcare Forum*, May/June 1986.

White, Jane K. "A Review of Organ Transplantation Policy." *Health Affairs*, Winter 1985.

Willging, Paul, Paul Kerschner, and Judith R. Peres. "Long-Term Care: The Malthusian Dilemma." *Health Care Financial Management*, December 1984.

Winston, William J. *Marketing Long-Term and Senior Care Services*. New York: Haworth Press, 1984.

"Women Provide 70 Percent of Free Home Health Care for Elderly." *Modern Healthcare*, August 29, 1986.

Yokle, Albin J. "Long-Term Care: The View Ahead." *Nursing Homes*, September/ October 1984.

Zapka, Jane G., Randy Schwartz, and Barbara Giloth. *Locating Resources for Evaluation*. Chicago: American Hospital Association, August 1982.

Index